THE GENETIC BASIS
FOR HUMAN DISEASE

M 948

FUNDAMENTAL AND CLINICAL ASPECTS OF INTERNAL MEDICINE
A Series of Volumes for the Postgraduate Course

THE UNIVERSITY OF MIAMI SCHOOL OF MEDICINE
Department of Internal Medicine
Coordinators
Jose S. Bocles, M.D.
William J. Harrington, M.D.

PUBLISHED

CLINICAL RHEUMATOLOGY
JOHN H. TALBOTT, M.D., EDITOR

MEDICAL ONCOLOGY
Howard E. Lessner, M.D., Editor

THE GENETIC BASIS FOR HUMAN DISEASE
Karl H. Muench, M.D.

FUNDAMENTAL AND CLINICAL ASPECTS OF INTERNAL MEDICINE
A Series of Volumes for the Postgraduate Course

THE GENETIC BASIS FOR HUMAN DISEASE

Karl H. Muench, M.D.

THE UNIVERSITY OF MIAMI SCHOOL OF MEDICINE
Department of Medicine

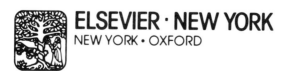
ELSEVIER · NEW YORK
NEW YORK · OXFORD

616.071
m948

Elsevier North-Holland, Inc.
52 Vanderbilt Avenue, New York, New York 10017

Distributors outside the United States and Canada:
Thomond Books
(A Division of Elsevier/North-Holland Scientific Publishers, Ltd)
P.O. Box 85
Limerick, Ireland

Library of Congress Cataloging in Publication Data

Muench, Karl H
  The genetic basis for human disease.

  (Fundamental and clinical aspects of internal
medicine)
    Bibliography: p.
    Includes index.
    1. Medical genetics.   2. Human genetics.
I. Title. II. Series.
RB155.M83   616.07'1'015751   78-31630
ISBN 0-444-00306-1
ISBN 0-444-00307-X (pbk.)

MANUFACTURED IN THE UNITED STATES OF AMERICA

DESIGNED BY LORETTA LI

To Any

CONTENTS

GENERAL PREFACE

Several years ago the Department of Internal Medicine of the University of Miami School of Medicine inaugurated an annual series of postgraduate courses entitled "Fundamental and Clinical Aspects of Internal Medicine." The first course, prompted by many requests from area physicians and medical societies, was timed to precede by one to two weeks the initial recertification examination of the American Board of Internal Medicine.

Among the teaching materials developed for this course was a group of booklets designed to follow closely the lecture presentations of subject matter judged to be of most pertinence to internists qualified for certification. Since the course was intensive and of only two weeks duration, we realized that the material to be presented had to be carefully selected, with assumptions made concerning content presumed to be already well known and also concerning material that would not in our judgment be needed by a competent general internist, although of great importance to the subspecialist.

The course has now been given each of the past four years. Its quality has been widely noted, and many physicians both from the United States and other countries have become annual registrants. Accordingly, it was felt that the course booklets might find a wider appeal if they were professionally produced and distributed by a publisher. This objective has been concluded by an agreement with Elsevier North-Holland to publish the series of volumes.

It should be stressed that these volumes are not intended to be comprehensive. They will not cover subject matter in the breadth ordinarily found in standard textbooks, but rather will supplement standard works. In order to be useful for the review course, the books will be inexpensive, and will be updated periodically, to maintain currency with advances in their respective areas.

We acknowledge the immeasurable help of our staff coordinator, Mrs. Arlene Gunn, and the secretarial staff of the divisions who contributed in the preparation of these volumes.

JOSE S. BOCLES, M.D.
WILLIAM J. HARRINGTON, M.D.

PREFACE TO THIS VOLUME

In light of the burden of genetic disease and the need for physicians of all specialties to refresh their reserves of genetic knowledge, I here provide a compact review of some basic principles of genetics, illustrated when possible by current clinical problems and research discoveries. In writing, I have assumed that the reader has had previous exposure to genetics. The material presented here is condensed to an extent appropriate only for a review. The presentation is not only condensed but necessarily incomplete. Areas such as immunogenetics, ecogenetics including pharmacogenetics, and ethical, legal, and social aspects of genetics are mentioned only briefly. Technical advances in prenatal diagnosis, such as amniocentesis with ultrasound localization and fetoscopy with fetal blood sampling, are left to specialized texts. References to genetic counseling are made throughout with no special section devoted to the practice of that art. Sources for further information in some of these areas are provided with the references in selected readings at the end of the book.

Whereas some areas are inadequately covered, others may appear to be unduly stressed or detailed. The selection reflects some of my own interests and also the exciting new findings in the current literature. Of necessity the balance is arbitrary to some extent. For better balance, the reader may refer to the several textbooks of genetics recommended in the general selected reading.

For brevity, I have largely omitted clinical descriptions of the diseases mentioned, although brief sketches appear in some of the figure legends. It is not my primary intention to review clinical aspects of the various diseases with which the reader has first-hand experience. For the purposes of this book, a listing of the physical findings in Down's syndrome, for example, is unnecessary. Rather, I wish to point out the ways in which various disorders illustrate genetic principles and the ways in which genetic mechanisms in turn illuminate the pathogenesis of disease. I wish to provide a framework for current understanding and for future data acquisition in genetic medicine.

I have omitted a formal glossary and have instead attempted to define genetic terms within the context of their appearances. An index serves to direct the reader to these definitions-in-context.

The chapter sequence may appear unorthodox and perhaps requires explanation. I begin with cytogenetics, because chromosomes are visible and familiar. They provide a tangible basis for the introduction of abstract concepts. Mendelian genetics is more easily grasped with chromosomes in mind. Historically, Mendelian genetics preceded knowledge of the biochemistry of the gene by more than half a century, and Mendelian genetics remains comprehensible without the details of genetic biochemistry. Therefore, I have placed the chapter "Mendelian Genetics" after "Cytogenetics" but before "Biochemistry of Genetic Expression." The chapter "Associations of Genetic Markers and Diseases" follows concepts of linkage and of Mendelian patterns developed in the preceding chapters. "Polygenic or Multifactorial Genetics" fits naturally at that point and still does not require biochemistry. With all of the foregoing in mind, the biochemistry of genetics is more understandable and fulfilling; thus the chapter "Biochemistry of Genetic Expression" is at this point rather than in a more traditional position at the beginning. The special area "Genetics and Cancer" is understandable only after some biochemical fundamentals have been presented. In my view the sections on cancer virology are appropriate because of the intricate relationships between viruses and the host genome. These interactions are involved in expression of malignancy in man, interactions best illustrated by the Epstein–Barr virus and Burkitt's lymphoma. The final chapter, "Treatment of Genetic Diseases," attempts to organize a framework, based on all of the preceding chapters, with which to place all current and future treatment in an orderly perspective. The chapter concludes with a brief discussion of genetic engineering.

Acknowledgments. Drawings are by Dr. Felix Soloni. Mrs. Barbara Pace typed (and retyped) the manuscript. Drs. William Awad, Julie Korenberg, Carol Shear, and Antero So critically read the manuscript or parts of it. Photographs were kindly provided by Drs. Lee Bricker, James Cleaver, Norman Gottlieb, Donald Harkness, Arthur Kornberg, Neal Penneys, W. B. Reed, Carol Shear, Marie Valdes-Dapena, Charles Vogel, and John Ziegler, and by Mr. and Mrs. Laurence Wiener. I thank them for their help.

Karl H. Muench, M.D.
Professor of Medicine
and Professor of Biochemistry
Chief of the Division of Genetic Medicine
University of Miami School of Medicine

THE NEED

Most physicians in the United States have had inadequate education in genetics. That fact is not surprising in view of the lack of formal courses in human genetics in medical schools at present, to say nothing of the past. Of 135 American and Canadian schools of medicine reporting course titles in descriptions of their curricula in the *1977–78 Curriculum Directory* of the Association of American Medical Colleges, only 67 (50%) list course titles including the word "genetics." These courses total an average of 24 hours. In comparison, courses in human sexuality are taught at 15 medical schools and total an average of 27 hours. (The comparison is interesting in the sense that human sexuality is required for human genetics!)

For physicians with premedical courses in genetics, the word elicits visions of fruit flies and mice. Other physicians think of genetics in terms of infants and children with debilitating genetic disorders, such as Down's syndrome or cystic fibrosis. However, more and more adult patients are asking genetic questions, and primary care physicians must now provide the answers, or sources, for medical and even for legal reasons.

Why is the demand for genetic information increasing? First, research is finding more and more diseases to be genetic or partially genetic in etiology, for example, cancer of the lung, the biggest killer among cancers, and porphyria cutanea tarda. Second, research is describing the biochemical mechanisms for diseases previously known to be genetic, for example, certain forms of gout. Third, advances in research are offering remedies if not genotypic cures for many genetic

1

disorders, and a whole new science of genetic engineering has grown up from the demonstration in 1972 that genes of one organism can be covalently bonded to genes of another organism. Fourth, mass encouragement of birth control and legalization of abortion has made planned parenthood much more of a reality and has engaged great public attention to genetic issues. Finally, the press is bombarding the public with speculative news stories concerning these dramatic advances in genetic issues.

The burden of genetic disorders is formidable. In 1976 it was estimated that 12 million Americans have a genetic disorder, and that life-years lost to such disorders are 6.5 times those lost to heart disease. It was further estimated that 30% of pediatric and 10% of adult hospital admissions are for genetic disorders.

Children with genetic disorders previously incompatible with normal adult life are now not only surviving but are marrying and having children. Examples are Wilson's disease and phenylketonuria. Adult patients with cystic fibrosis are no longer rare. These changes in age and reproductive patterns pose new problems for physicians primarily engaged in care of adults.

The primary physician will on occasion feel unable to answer genetic questions arising from clinical situations. Then his legal responsibility is to obtain or at least advise expert consultation. To locate American physicians who provide genetic counseling is more difficult than to locate other medical specialists, because clinical geneticists usually are not listed by specialty in local telephone books. The reason for this situation is that genetics is not one of the 69 clinical specialties recognized by the American Medical Association. In comparison, nutrition and hypnosis are recognized specialties, as is diabetes mellitus. (In this book, I shall discuss genetic aspects of the disorders called diabetes mellitus.) In Canada, the Canadian College of Medical Geneticists accredits holders of the PhD, MD, or DDS degrees who possess the necessary qualifications in medical genetics. Plans for an American body or similar accreditation are under discussion. The accessibility of American medical geneticists should increase with such accreditation and recognition of the accrediting body. A list of centers where genetic consultation is available is given in the International Directory of Genetic Services (ed 5. White Plains, NY, The National Foundation–March of Dimes, 1977).

What situations indicate genetic counseling, provided either by the primary physician or by a consulting geneticist? The recent discovery or known presence in the patient of

an anatomical defect present at birth
abnormal development of sexual organs, secondary sexual charac-
    teristics, sexual function, or fertility
repeated abortions or miscarriages
abnormal mental development
abnormal physical growth or stature
a chromosomal abnormality
a metabolic disease
any disease known to be inherited.

The same indications often apply when the inquirer is not affected but is a family member. Impending marriage, impending parenthood, or pregnancy itself sharpen concern. Particular indications in pregnancy are advanced age and exposure to drugs, radiation, and infection. Finally, consanguinity is an indication for premarital counseling.

Probably 90% of patients with these indications do not actually receive genetic counseling as a part of their care. Perhaps this review will help primary physicians to meet the obvious need.

CYTOGENETICS

THE HUMAN KARYOTYPE

The total number of single genes coding for the structural and enzymatic proteins in man is on the order of 50,000, and these are contained in DNA in 46 chromosomes in each diploid cell. The chromosomes are typically visualized in peripheral lymphocytes that have been placed in tissue culture, stimulated to divide, arrested in metaphase, and osmotically swelled to give a picture as in Figure 1. Chromosomes cut from such a picture are arranged in homologous pairs to give the familiar karyotype shown in Figure 2. Chromosomes in nondividing cells are not uniformly condensed and have only half the mass of these visible chromosomes, which have already doubled prior to cell division. Of the 23 chromosome pairs, 22 are autosomes, and one pair comprises the sex chromosomes: X and X in females, and X and Y in males. One member of each chromosome pair is maternal, the other member paternal in origin. The chromosomes are identifiable by their sizes, by the positions of their centromeres, and by their characteristic banding patterns after staining with conventional or fluorescent dyes. Thus, the chromosome pair 17 is distinguishable from the chromosome pair 18 by banding, even though these pairs are similar in size and both are submetacentric as shown in Figure 3.

MITOSIS AND MEIOSIS

During mitosis or somatic cell division, each chromosome first replicates to give the familiar structure with four arms or chromatids. Symmetric division distributes one copy to each of the identical, diploid,

4

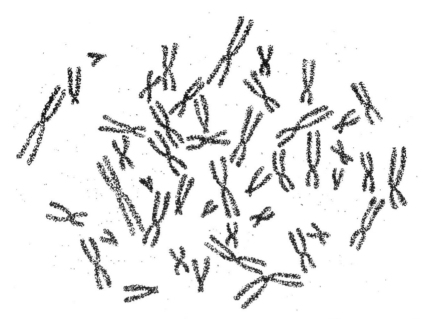

FIGURE 1. Human male chromosomes arrested in metaphase. The treatment of the cell in hypotonic buffer disperses the chromosomes. Each chromosome consists of two sister chromatids joined at the centromere. The diploid number of chromosomes in man is 46.

daughter cells, as shown in Figure 4. In contrast, division of germ cells to form haploid ova or sperm entails meiosis, in which the first, or reduction division, leads to segregation, one chromosome of each pair going to each daughter cell as shown in Figure 5. Segregation is in one sense the reverse of fertilization, which brings together one maternal and one paternal chromosome to form each pair in the zygote. The essence of Mendel's first law is that maternal and paternal chromosomes (or corresponding loci on maternal and paternal chromosomes) come together in fertilization and separate (segregate) in gametogenesis, specifically in the reduction division of meiosis. However, any given gamete contains a random, independent assortment of maternal and paternal chromosomes, and that random assortment is the essence of Mendel's second law.

The independent assortment of chromosomes during meiosis is a major reason for the variation of the genetic constitution in different

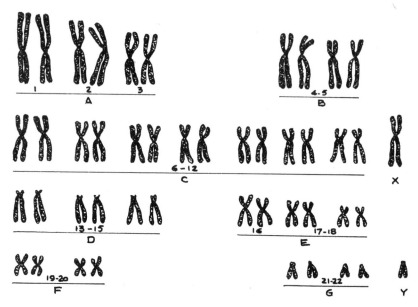

FIGURE 2. Chromosomes cut from a photograph of a preparation as in Fig. 1 are arranged in seven groups, A to G, according to size. Within each group chromosomes are arranged by position of the centromere. The X and Y chromosomes are difficult to distinguish from those of groups C and G, respectively, and members of groups, B, C, D, F, and G are usually indistinguishable without banding patterns.

individuals. Each gamete has 2^{23} (8 million) possible combinations of chromosomes from the 23 pairs, and each set of parents has $2^{23} \times 2^{23} = 7 \times 10^{13}$ possible chromosome combinations to offer the children.

The Y chromosome is unique in that it precisely derives from the paternal lineage. The Y chromosome bears only one known gene, that for H–Y antigen, the primary determinant of male gonadal sex.

CROSSING OVER

Even more variation is provided by breakage, exchange, and rejoining of chromosomes. This process occurs between homologous chromatids during meiosis and is called crossing over, shown in Figure 6. The crossover forms a chiasma, and the chiasmata in a meiotic preparation can be counted under the microscope. In crossing over, an allele at a

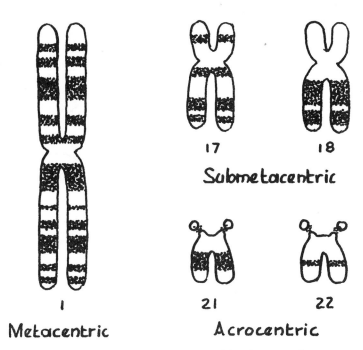

17   18

Submetacentric

21   22

1

Metacentric   Acrocentric

FIGURE 3. Variation in size and centromere position (acrocentric, metacentric) seen in human chromosomes. Idealized, composite banding patterns are shown for chromosomes 17 and 18 and for chromosomes 21 and 22; these chromosomes would otherwise be indistinguishable. Here the acrocentric chromosomes have satellites, chromatin separated from the main chromosome by poorly staining decondensed chromatin. The basis for different banding patterns is not understood.

gene locus on one chromatid is exchanged for an allele in the corresponding locus on a homologous chromatid. This recombination provides segregation of alleles at linked loci. The four gametic products of a single crossover event are two recombinants and two nonrecombinants. Genes on the same chromosome are called syntenic. Crossing over is so frequent that genes on opposite ends of long chromosomes segregate independently.

Crossing over of sister chromatids (sister chromatid exchange) occurs during mitosis in somatic cells, but the reason for this event in somatic cells is not understood.

The random reassortment of alleles produces an incomprehensible number of different gametes. Even if we conservatively assume only

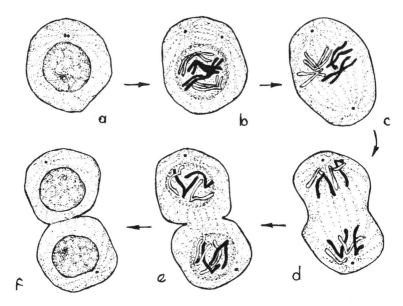

FIGURE 4. Mitosis. For clarity only two of the 23 human chromosome pairs are shown. In going from (a) to (b) each chromosome has replicated itself and has condensed to give the characteristic sister chromatids joined at the centromere as seen in metaphase (c). The replicated chromosomes then divide in going from (c) to (d), and each daughter cell (f) has the original diploid chromosome constitution and DNA content of the mother cell (a).

10,000 genes, only 10% difference in maternal and paternal alleles, and only one crossover per chromosome, a single human donor could produce 6×10^{43} different gametes. The lifetime production of spermatozoa (10^{12}) and ova (400) are only infinitesimal fractions of the possibilities. Thus, with the incomplete exception of monovular twins, every person is genetically unique throughout all history, past and future.

MAPPING OF GENES ON CHROMOSOMES

When two gene loci reside on different chromosome pairs, they segregate independently in meiosis, and the probability is 0.5 that a specified allele at one of the two loci will occur in gamete with a specified allele at the other locus. This probability of 0.5 results from total in-

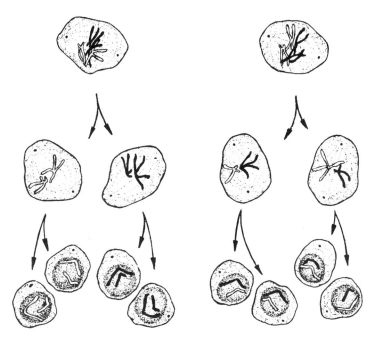

FIGURE 5. Meiosis. Again, only two chromosome pairs are shown. The members of each pair segregate during the first, or reduction, division. Independent assortment of the chromosomes in this reduction division gives four (2^2) possible combinations for two chromosome pairs, as shown in the middle of the diagram. For 23 chromosome pairs, the number of possible combinations is 2^{23}, 8.4 million. In the second meiotic division, the replicated chromosomes split as in mitosis to give gametes with a haploid chromosome constitution, one chromosome from each original pair.

dependence or nonlinkage of the loci. Correspondingly, gene loci juxtaposed on the same chromosome segregate together and have a recombination fraction of 0 unless there is a crossover at a site between them. The probability that such crossing over will occur is a direct function of the distance between the loci, or where they "map." Thus, the recombination fraction varies from 0 to 0.5 and is the measure of the crossover probability. When two loci have a recombination fraction of 0.01 they are a genetic map distance of 1 centiMorgan (cM) apart. The actual physical distance between loci does not precisely correspond to the recombination fraction, although agreement is close for low values of the recombination fraction. At higher values corre-

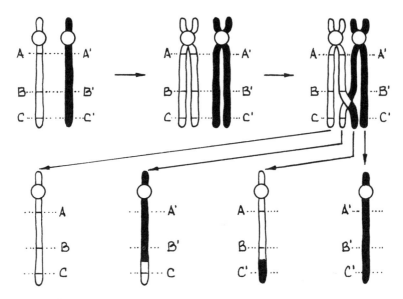

FIGURE 6. Crossing over occurs during pairing in meiosis. In this diagram each chromosome first replicates; then homologous chromatids break, exchange, and rejoin to give two recombinant and two nonrecombinant gametes. The letter pairs, for example A and A', are alleles, two of several possible variations of a gene occurring at one locus.
Adapted from Stern C: Principles of Human Genetics, ed. 3. San Francisco, WH Freeman & Co, 1973.

spondence decreases, because measurable crossovers or recombinations are less than expected for the larger physical map distances. The decrease results because double crossovers are more likely to occur at the larger distances, and double crossovers negate the recombinants formed from single crossovers between the same two loci.

In human testicular biopsies, the number of chiasmata (crossovers) seen on the 22 autosomal pairs averages about 52. Because a crossover produces equal numbers of recombinant and nonrecombinant gametes, each crossover represents a recombination fraction of 0.5 and a map distance of 50 cM. Therefore, the total genetic length of the haploid genome in man is about $52 \times 50 = 2600$ cM. A large chromosome of perhaps 200 cM would then provide ample opportunity for crossing over, given the value of 50 cM per crossover. (The recombination frequency may be as much as 50% greater in females than in males, for reasons not understood.)

Gene-mapping information comes from two types of studies. The first, or linkage studies, tell us how close loci are to each other in a linkage group without localizing them to a specific chromosome. The second type of study designates on which chromosome a gene resides, thereby linking it or mapping it with the other genes on the same chromosome. Figure 7 shows the gene map of chromosome 1. Pedigree analysis is one way to determine linkage. For example, consider a woman who is a double heterozygote for color blindness and glucose-6-phosphate dehydrogenase (G6PD) deficiency, as shown in Figure 8. In this case, both loci are known to be on the X chromosome by family studies. We may ask how far apart are the loci. The mutant alleles may both be on the same X chromosome (in coupling) or one may be on the paternally derived X chromosome and the other on the maternally derived X chromosome (in repulsion). Examination of the

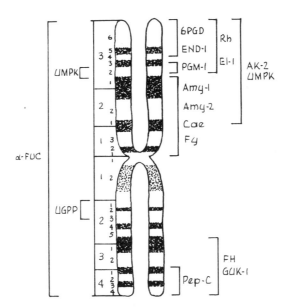

FIGURE 7. Gene map of chromosome 1. The loci for the several genes indicated are now mapped to chromosome 1. For example, the Fy (Duffy blood group) is on the proximal and El-1 (elliptocytosis-1) is on the distal part of the short arm (q), and Pep-C (peptidase-C) is on the distal extremity of the long arm (p).

Adapted from deGrouchy J. Turleau C: Clinical Atlas of Human Chromosomes. New York, John Wiley & Sons, 1977.

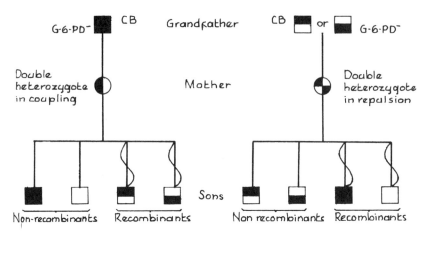

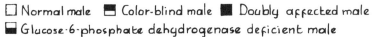

□ Normal male   ■ Color-blind male   ■ Doubly affected male
■ Glucose-6-phosphate dehydrogenase deficient male

FIGURE 8. Loci for color blindness and G6PD deficiency may reside on the same or on homologous X chromosomes in carrier females ("Mother" here). Examination of their fathers ("Grandfather" here) provides the answer, as shown in this diagram. Numbers of recombinant and nonrecombinant sons then provide the data base for map distance between the loci.

Adapted from McKusick VA, Ruddle FH: The status of the gene map of the human chromosomes. Science 196:390, 1977.

woman's father provides the answer, and study of the sons of many such women gives a value for the recombination fraction. For example, if a father is both color blind and a G6PD variant, then the loci are in coupling on the paternal X chromosome, and all of the sons of his daughters are affected unless recombination occurs. When ten such families were studied, one in 20 sons was a recombinant. The data translate directly into map distance between the loci. Thus the genes for color blindness and G6PD have a recombination fraction of 0.05 and are roughly 5 cM apart in their linkage group, the X chromosome.

When only a single sibship is available for study, the likelihood of an observed association of two alleles at different values of the recombination fraction can be compared to the likelihood of that association if the alleles were not linked, that is, if the recombination fraction were 0.5. The log of the ratio of those likelihoods is a lod score (for "log of the odds") and provides evidence for or against linkage. Moreover, the lod score indicates the degree of linkage, or map distance, because selected test values for recombination fraction produce a range of lod scores with a maximum at the recombination fraction closest to the actual value. An example is given in Figure 9.

Sometimes direct evidence for tight gene linkage comes from observation of gene products such as the hemoglobins Lepore, which result from unequal crossing over of neighboring β and δ globin genes.

The fact that more genes (more than 100) have been assigned to the X chromosome than to any autosome is a direct consequence of observations made possible by the different sex chromosome constitution

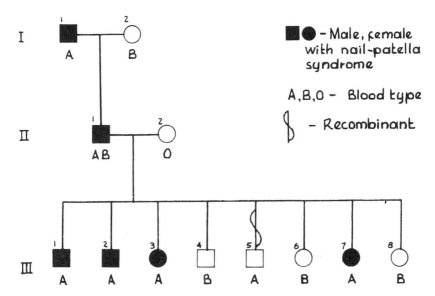

FIGURE 9. The loci for ABO blood group and for nail-patella syndrome are both on chromosome 9. As seen from his parents' phenotypes, person II-1 in this pedigree has the blood group A allele and the nail–patella allele on the same chromosome 9 (in coupling) and the blood group B allele and the normal allele of the nail–patella locus on the other chromosome 9. Of his eight children, only one (III-5) is a recombinant, and the recombination fraction from this one sibship is $1/8 = 0.12$. Therefore, the loci are about 12 cM apart. If the grandparents (I-1 and I-2) were unavailable for study, the linkage phase in II-1 would be unknown, but the method of lods could be applied for the III sibship of 7 and 1. The method gives a lod score maximal at 0.787 for the recombination fraction 0.10, odds of 6 to 1 that the loci are linked about 10 cM apart. Odds of 1000 to 1 are taken as strong evidence for linkage and are obtainable by combining data from mutiple pedigrees.

Adapted from McKusick VA, Ruddle FH: The status of the gene map of the human chromosomes. Science 196:390, 1977.

of males and females. Assignment of single genes or of linkage groups to specific autosomes is more difficult but is yielding to new methods, and more than 110 assignments have been made. The classical example is segregation of Duffy blood-group substance with a morphological marker on chromosome 1.

Interspecies somatic cell hybridization is a powerful new method in which human cells are fused with mouse cells, for example, in tissue culture. The resulting human–murine hybrid cells are grown in a medium that selects against the original mouse and human cells. The hybrid cells randomly lose human chromosomes during subsequent cell divisions. Ultimately, stable clones containing one or a few human chromosomes are assayed for presence of the human gene products under study. A simple matching of presence or absence of the gene product with presence or absence of a given chromosome allows assignment of genes to chromosomes. Variations of the method allow localizations of genes to parts of chromosomes fragmented by ionizing radiation or to parts of chromosomes carried as stable translocations in certain families.

More than 210 loci have now been mapped, and linkage groups are known for every human chromosome except Y. This information can be used not only in premorbid diagnosis but in prenatal diagnosis of disorders for which no direct enzyme assay exists. Thus hemophilia has been detected before birth by linkage with glucose-6-phosphate dehydrogenase (G6PD). In this case, crossovers producing recombinants occur in only 5% of gametes, and prenatal diagnosis is 95% accurate, a figure much better than the 50% accuracy of prenatal diagnosis based on sex determination.

MUTATIONS

If the chromatids break at different points before reunion, unequal crossing over results. Unequal crossing over may give rise to gene duplication, or, reciprocally, gene deletion, both of which are varieties of mutation. The inequality may be smaller than a gene and lead to deletions or additions of single codons or even single bases, as exemplified by several of the hemoglobinopathies. Crossing over can occur in the middle of nonallelic genes to give, for example, the combined δ–β hemoglobin subunit observed in hemoglobin Lepore or δ–β in anti-Lepore. The process of gene duplication encourages diversity through evolution by allowing one member of the two identical new genes to mutate at random while its essential function continues to be served by the other gene. Genes for closely similar proteins are often found to be linked, probably because they arose by gene duplication. For example, in man there are two genes for the α chain of hemoglobin, and there are two genes for γ chains that differ by a single amino acid.

Other varieties of mutation occurring during the process of meiosis include gene inversion, in which a segment of chromatid turns through 180° before reunion; and translocation, in which a chromatid detached from one chromosome is rejoined to another chromosome. Balanced, reciprocal translocations are tolerated in the somatic cell line, but in the germ cell line may produce abnormal gametes containing extra or deficient chromosomal parts after meiosis. The resultant zygotes have multiple defects, often resulting in spontaneous abortion. Couples with this problem typically ask for counseling after several first-trimester abortions.

NONDISJUNCTION OF CHROMOSOMES

Nondisjunction is the failure of chromosomes to separate during division, one daughter cell containing an extra chromosome missing from the other daughter cell, as shown in Figure 10. During gametogenesis

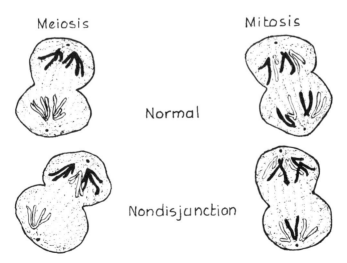

FIGURE 10. Nondisjunction can occur in meiosis or in mitosis and can involve autosomes or sex chromosomes.

such nondisjunction of autosome 21 leads to trisomy 21 or Down's syndrome, and nondisjunction of the sex chromosomes causes Turner's (XO) syndrome, Klinefelter's syndrome (XXY), and the XYY male. Recently, the XYY male has been a focus of debate in a controversial area of human behavioral genetics. The consensus is that XYY males have slightly lowered intelligence as a group but are not predisposed to excessive criminal or aggressive behavior. Visible chromosomal defects seen in these and other syndromes are common, being observed in about 1% of all live births. About one third of all zygotes are aborted spontaneously, and about one third of these have chromosomal defects. The frequency of XO in abortuses is so high (20 to 30%) that an estimated 2 to 2.5% of all concepti are XO. Less than 5% of these survive to be born alive, a curious fact in view of the good survival of Turner's syndrome patients after birth. Figure 11 shows a child with Turner's syndrome.

In Down's syndrome (Figure 12) and in the other autosomal trisomies, there is a prominent maternal age effect: The frequency of autosomal nondisjunction in the maturing ovum increases with the age of the mother (Figure 13). The effect is not seen in spermatogenesis in the aging father even though paternal nondisjunction may be responsible for any given case of Down's syndrome. One study revealed a paternal source for the extra chromosome 21 in 24% (31/129) of the cases.

Possibly the maternal age effect results from differences between oogenesis and spermatogenesis. Spermatogonia each produce four spermatids in a 64-day process repeating from puberty and lasting for life. In contrast, oogonia propagate during fetal life but stop at about six months' gestation. At birth each female has about 750,000 oocytes. These have completed the chromosomal doubling for the first meiotic division, but remain in an arrested state until ovulation, when the reduction division is completed. The equational division occurs after penetration of the ovum by a spermatozoon. One ovum and two or three polar bodies are the products of the meiotic divisions in the female. Perhaps the prolonged dormancy of the oocyte in the prophase of the meiotic reduction division renders the oocyte vulnerable to nondisjunction.

The increase in Down's syndrome progeny born to mothers over 35 is striking, and for this reason diagnostic amniocentesis should be considered for the estimated 300,000 American women each year who are

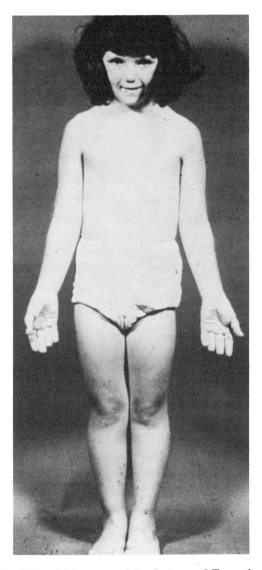

FIGURE 11. This child exhibits some of the features of Turner's syndrome, including short stature, triangular face with hypoplastic mandible, pterygium colli, broad chest, and cubitus valgus. Ovarian agenesis leads to primary amenorrhea and absence of puberty. The phenotype is variable, and the diagnosis may be missed until adolescence. Mild mental retardation may be present, but normal or even high intelligence can be attained. Cardiovascular and renal malformations may be silent and should be searched for. Coarctation of the aorta occurs in more than half of the cases. Estrogen therapy usually induces development of internal and external genitalia, secondary sexual characteristics, and menses.

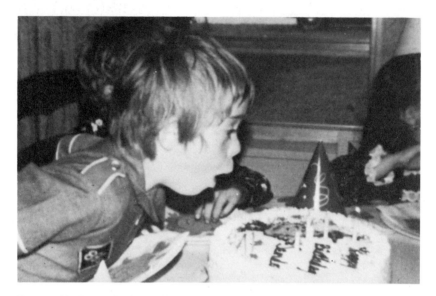

FIGURE 12. Often children with Down's syndrome can fully integrate into family life. This boy competed successfully in school and at play, socializing well with children two years younger. I am including this picture to balance the usual textbook picture of Down's syndrome and to modulate the often reflex insistence by physicians to institutionalize such children at birth.

pregnant and over 35. The United States Public Health Service has endorsed amniocentesis for this group. That endorsement certainly raises legal issues concerning the obligation of physicians to inform their patients of the amniocentesis option. The matter is complicated by lack of sufficient laboratories to perform the karyotyping.

In recent years the average age of mothers of infants with Down's syndrome has moved downward worldwide. As a result accurate age-based risk figures are unavailable.

TRANSLOCATION DOWN'S SYNDROME

Most cases of Down's syndrome result from nondisjunction and are, therefore, sporadic. That is, they are genetic, but not inherited, and unaffected family members cannot transmit the disease to progeny. But occasional cases result from translocation between chromosome

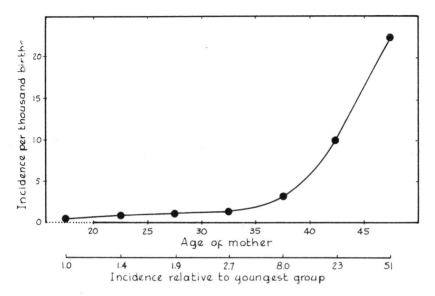

FIGURE 13. The effect of maternal age on the incidence of Down's syndrome underlines the importance of karyotyping affected infants and particularly younger mothers.

Adapted from Stern C: Principles of Human Genetics, ed. 3. San Francisco, WH Freeman & Co, 1973.

21 and another chromosome, usually 14 as shown in Figure 14. These cases are hereditary and should be searched for by karyotyping, especially in young mothers of infants with Down's syndrome. About 10% of such infants born to mothers under 30 have translocation Down's syndrome. In about one half of the cases of translocation Down's syndrome, the parents have normal karyotypes, the translocation being new in the affected child, but in the other one half, one parent carries a translocation chromosome.

Nondisjunction taking place during mitosis in the zygote rather than during meiosis of gametogenesis gives rise to mosaics such as the complementary XO/XXX. In the same way individuals may be mosaics for Down's syndrome with intermediate phenotype. About one half of patients with Turner's syndrome are not XO but are either mosaics or have a structural abnormality such as an isochromosome of the X chromosome. An isochromosome is a symmetrical chromosome consisting of two long arms or two short arms and resulting from "horizontal" instead of "vertical" division of a chromosome.

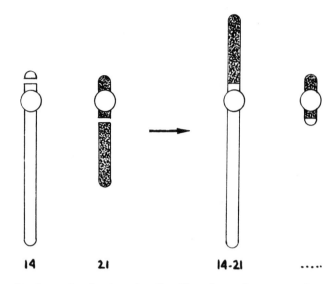

14   21   14-21   .....

FIGURE 14. A carrier for translocation Down's syndrome may have a 14–21 chromosome resulting from breaks in the short arm of chromosome 14 and in the long arm of chromosome 21 with rejoining as shown in this diagram. The small chromosome composed of the reciprocal fragments is presumably lost.
Adapted from Stern C: Principles of Human Genetics., ed. 3. San Francisco, WH Freeman & Co., 1973.

CHROMOSOME GAIN AND LOSS

The loss of an autosome is almost always lethal. However, partial loss of an autosome, for example, the deletion of the short arm of chromosome 5 in cri-du-chat syndrome, may be compatible with life. Conversely, the presence of an extra autosome (trisomy) is sometimes tolerated, at least for chromosomes 13 (Patau's syndrome), 18 (Edward's syndrome), and 21, (Down's syndrome); and trisomy 21 occurs with the relatively high frequency of one in 500 live births. Extra sex chromosomes are compatible with life, as in Klinefelter's syndrome (one in 500 male births), XYY males, and XXX females (one in 800 female births). A single X chromosome is present in Turner's syndrome. Viability in this special case of monosomy is perhaps understandable, since normal males have only one X chromosome and since one X chromosome is inactive in every normal female somatic cell. However, the "inactive" X chromosome must have some function, because normal females and XO females clearly differ.

THE LYON PHENOMENON

If both X chromosomes remained active for the lifetime of the zygote, then the proteins encoded by genes in the X chromosomes would potentially occur in double dosage in females and in single dosage in males. In the Lyon phenomenon, one X chromosome in every cell of the early female embryo is inactivated randomly and forms the Barr body (Figure 15) seen in interphase nuclei. The Barr bodies may be visualized in stained smears of buccal mucosal cells or in the accessory nuclear lobes, "drumsticks," of neutrophiles in Wright-stained blood smears. (Quinacrine staining reveals a fluorescent Y chromosome in nuclei of about two thirds of buccal mucosal cells from normal males. Cells from XYY males frequently have two such bodies.) Once the random inactivation has occurred, the same X chromosome is the inactive one in all of the descendent cells. The only cells excepted from this process are the primordial germ cells. Females who are heterozygous for an enzyme coded on the X chromosome, for example, glucose-6-phosphate dehydrogenase (G6PD), are mosaics with wild-type enzymes carried by approximately one half of their cells and mutant enzymes carried by the other half.

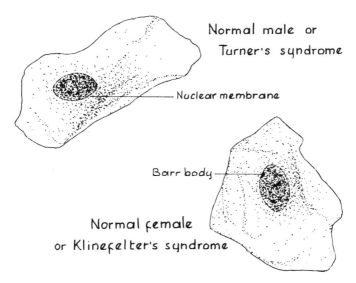

FIGURE 15. The inactive X chromosome is often visible as a Barr body in the interphase nucleus. Epithelial cells scraped from the buccal mucosa are seen here.

MENDELIAN GENETICS

*If the features of the countenance, the
outside of the body, are often hereditary,
why not also the inside?*

Dr. William Cadogan, 1771

GENES AND PHENOTYPES

In the Mendelian sense, a gene is the unit of inheritance responsible
for the presence of a given genetic characteristic. The pairing of the
chromosomes is consistent with the fact that each zygote contains a
gene on each chromosome at a single locus. The two genes carried by
a single individual at a given locus on a chromosomal pair constitute
that person's genotype and may be identical or may differ. Differing
genes at the same locus are called alleles. If the genes at a locus are
identical, the individual is homozygous at that locus. An individual
with different alleles at a locus is heterozygous at that locus. During
normal meiosis, alleles segregate, one going to each gamete. Whereas
an individual carries only one or two alleles at one locus, other possible
alleles may exist in the gene pool of the population. Loci with multiple
alleles that are maintained at frequencies above 1% in the gene pool
are called polymorphic.

We now recognize the existence of many polymorphisms in the human population, largely because of evidence obtained by electropho-
resis of enzymes. In a series of proteins examined for electrophoretic
variability in normal human beings and other species, about 30% of
the proteins show variability. The number is a minimal figure for true
variation, because changes from an amino acid residue to another of

22

like charge does not produce electrophoretic variability. For example, the change from a negatively charged glutamate residue to a neutral valine residue in sickle cell hemoglobin produces electrophoretic difference, but a change to an aspartate residue, also negative, does not.

The phenotype denotes the recognizable characteristic determined by the genotype. Differing genotypes may present the same phenotype. For example, the homozygous genotype, *AA*, may appear identical to the heterozygous genotype, *Aa*. With respect to the heterozygote, *Aa*, if the phenotype is identical to that of the homozygote, *AA*, then the phenotype of *A* is dominant and the phenotype of *a* is recessive. The terms *dominant* and *recessive* describe the phenotype, not the genotype. Thus, even a mutant gene producing no protein product at all can present a dominant phenotype.

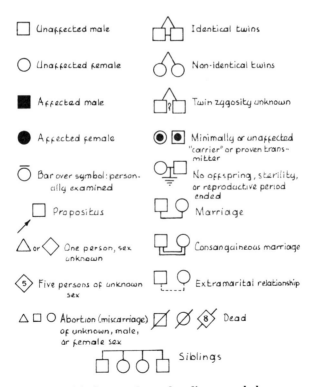

FIGURE 16. Commonly used pedigree symbols.

Given a patient with a characteristic phenotype, we can determine its mode of inheritance by pedigree analysis. The mode of inheritance gives information concerning the character of the disease, even the underlying biochemistry. Any disease inherited in one of the Mendelian patterns is caused by a defect in a single protein regardless of the diversity of phenotypic manifestations. The precise mode of inheritance provides an important clue concerning the type of defective gene product: enzyme or structural protein.

AUTOSOMAL RECESSIVE INHERITANCE

About 1000 autosomal recessive genetic disorders have been described. The classical pedigree (Figure 17) shows only the progeny of a single marriage involved, children of both sexes affected, and the ratio of affected to unaffected children, 1:3. The parents are pheno-

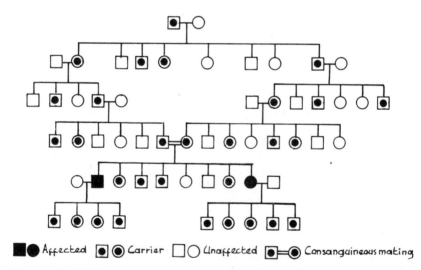

FIGURE 17. Idealized pedigree of an autosomal recessive trait. The heterozygous carriers are ordinarily not evident but are often detectable by specific biochemical assays. The precise ratios of affected, carrier, and unaffected progeny given for each mating here for purposes of illustration must not obscure the independence of probabilities for each sibling in reality.

typically normal. The appearance of the disease in a single generation of a pedigree gives a horizontal pattern. For rare autosomal recessive traits, increased consanguinity can be demonstrated in affected families, a finding indicative of recessive transmission.

Disorders caused by enzyme defects are generally inherited in the recessive mode. Deficient activity of a specific enzyme has been demonstrated in more than 170 disorders. All classical Garrodian metabolic defects are recessive. This is understandable, because the levels of most enzymes in living cells are not limiting; the heterozygote with half the normal enzyme level is ordinarily capable of synthesizing the particular product in an amount sufficient for a normal phenotype. This concept is illustrated by Figure 18, showing the pathway of synthesis of F. The initial substrate, A, may have multiple sources and roles in

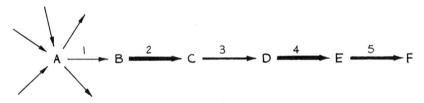

FIGURE 18. The metabolic pathway for biosynthesis of F from A. The thicknesses of arrows indicate relative activities of the five numbered enzymes.

other pathways, but, once converted to B, the only end product is F. This first, committed step is classically the rate-limiting step in conversion of A into F, and its enzyme, 1, is the site for feedback control. In contrast, enzymes 2, 3, 4, and 5 are present in surplus and would be sufficient for the pathway even if decreased in amount or activity by a factor of two. The heterozygosity of both parents is, of course, characteristic of autosomal recessive inheritance and can be proven in many cases by direct enzyme assays.

Homozygous enzyme deficiency results in disease by various patterns that a block may produce: accumulation of the substrate before the block, starvation for product F, compensation by excessive activity of enzyme 1, and new pathways for the intermediates before the block. Consequences differ for catabolic and anabolic pathways.

Usually the complete presentation of a disease is readily comprehensible from the fundamental enzyme defect and its attendant, initial metabolic disorder. Sometimes, however, the connection is less clear.

For example, children with absent adenosine deaminase have severe combined immunodeficiency, with both T-cell and B-cell function greatly impaired. The mechanism by which this enzyme deficit produces immunodeficiency is unknown.

Almost all enzyme defects are characterized by an absence or by a decrease in enzyme activity. An exception is primary elevation of 5-phosphoribosyl-1-pyrophosphate (PRPP) synthetase activity, leading to purine overproduction and gout. In this exceptional enzymopathy, inheritance is autosomal dominant. The dominant inheritance pattern is directly consequential from the enzymatic lesion: a structural alteration in PRPP synthetase causes the enzyme to have a higher maximal rate of catalysis. Therefore, even a single dose of the mutant allele causes higher PRPP production. PRPP is a substrate for the amido transferase, which catalyzes the first committed step in de novo purine synthesis. The rate of the amido transferase in vivo is determined by the PRPP concentration, because PRPP is present in limiting amounts. Therefore, the increased availability of PRPP leads to increased purine production and ultimately, gout.

Mutations in enzymes can lead to increased activity in other ways. In the Hektoen variant of human G6PD, the substitution of a tyrosine for a histidine residue because of a single point mutation leads to overproduction of the enzyme with consequent fourfold increase in its activity in red and white blood cells.

Perhaps the best known example of autosomal dominant inheritance associated with overactivity of an enzyme is acute intermittent porphyria, in which overactivity of δ-amino levulinic acid (ALA) synthetase leads to the overproduction of ALA and porphobilinogen, a characteristic of this disease. Here the enzyme is at the control point, the first committed step in a metabolic pathway with no branch points and a single final product (heme in this case). Such enzymes are subject to control by inhibition, by repression, or both, as in this case. A point mutation could cause insensitivity of the enzyme to an inhibitor or insensitivity of the gene to a repressor. Either mechanism would give a dominant pattern of inheritance. However, uroporphyrinogen synthetase, the enzyme that acts on porphobilinogen in the heme pathway, has only 50% of normal activity in patients with acute intermittent porphyria, and the overactivity of ALA synthetase also can be explained by a resultant diminution of heme to act as a feedback regulator.

HARDY-WEINBERG LAW

The gene frequencies in a population can be calculated easily if the gene products are identifiable. For example, alleles on chromosome 2 determine the MN blood type. If both alleles are M, the phenotype is M and the genotype is MM. Other possible genotypes are MN and NN. In a population of 1000 people typed for MN we might find

				TOTAL
Phenotype	M	MN	N	
Genotype	MM	MN	NN	
Number of people	370	480	150	1000
Number of M genes	740	480	0	1220
Number of N genes	0	480	300	780
Total number of genes				2000

Therefore, the gene frequency of M is 1220/2000 or 0.61, and the gene frequency of N is 780/2000 or 0.39.

With these figures for gene frequencies we can test the assumptions that mating in the generation preceding this population was random with respect to MN blood type and that survival was not affected by MN blood type. Did the preceding generation have the same gene frequencies? Each gamete carries one allele, either M or N. Assume that for the preceding generation 0.61 of gametes carried M and that 0.39 of gametes carried N, as is the case for the sample population. Then the probability for zygotes of genotype MM would have been $(0.61)(0.61) = 0.372$, and 372 of the sample population would have that genotype. The figure expected on the basis of the assumption agrees well with the observed figure of 370. Similarly, the probability for zygotes of genotype NN would have been $(0.39)(0.39) = 0.152$. In close agreement, 150 of the sample population have that genotype. Finally, the probability for zygotes of genotype MN would have been the difference, $1 - 0.372 - 0.152 = 0.476$, in good agreement with the 480 actually observed in the population of 1000. Thus the sample population is in genetic equilibrium, with random mating and survival unaffected by these alleles. These observations are generalized in the Hardy–Weinberg Law, demonstrated independently by an English mathematician and a German physician in 1908. Thus, if there are two alleles at a given locus with gene frequencies p and q, then $p + q =$

1, and the distribution of people with the possible genotypes pp, pq, and qq is expressed by the binomial expansion, $(p+q)^2 = 1 = p^2 + 2pq + q^2$. Now we shall see what this law tells us about autosomal recessive diseases and their stable frequencies in populations.

Cystic fibrosis is the most common autosomal recessive disease of white Americans, 4% of whom are heterozygotes. For every homozygote with a recessive disease, there are many heterozygous carriers, and the rarer the disease the greater is the disproportion, as shown by

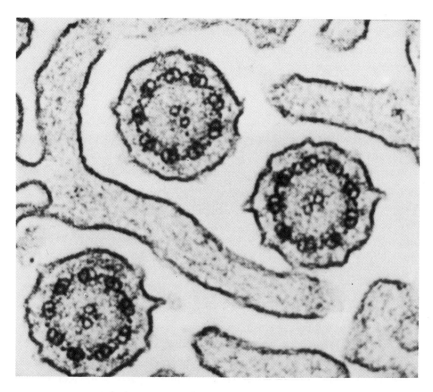

FIGURE 19. Immotile-cilia syndrome. An adult male with a history of sterility and chronic lung disease may have cystic fibrosis. Another autosomal recessive disease to be considered in the differential diagnosis is immotile-cilia syndrome, in which many patients exhibit Kartagener's triad: bronchiectasis, sinusitis, and situs inversus. This electron micrograph of nasal epithelium shows three cilia in cross section, each with a different orientation of the two central microtubules. This and other abnormalities of the microtubules render sperm immotile in this syndrome.

From Eliasson R, Mossberg B, Camner P, Afzelius BA: The immotile cilia syndrome. N Engl J Med 297:1–6, 1977.

the Hardy–Weinberg law for random mating: Let q = the proportion of cystic fibrosis genes in the population and let p = the proportion of normal alleles. Then $p + q = 1$, and the binomial distribution, $(p+q)^2 = p^2 + 2pq + q^2 = 1$, describes the distribution of normal homozygotes, heterozygotes, and affected homozygotes. The frequency of cystic fibrosis in the population (q^2) is 1/2500. Therefore, the gene frequency or proportion of abnormal alleles (q) is 1/50, and the proportion of normal alleles (p) is 49/50. Therefore, the frequency of heterozygotes or carriers in the population ($2pq$) is 98/2500 or 4%. There are 98 carriers for every afflicted homozygote. In the rarer recessive diseases the discrepancy between the numbers of identifiable homozygotes and of carriers becomes much greater. Thus for one form of albinism occurring in one of 40,000 persons $q = 1/200$, $p = 199/200$ and $2pq = 398/40,000$. There are 398 carriers for every identifiable homozygote, and 1% of the population are carriers for this disease. For Wilson's disease about 0.5% of the population are carriers, 1000 for every afflicted homozygote.

Why is consanguinity often found in pedigrees of recessive disease? If one person in 200 carries Wilson's disease (Figure 20), then the chance for random mates to have afflicted children is 1/200 × 1/200 × 1/4 or one in 160,000 for each pregnancy. However, if the mates are first cousins (having 1/8 genes in common) then the chance for affected children is 1/200 × 1/8 × 1/4 or one in 6400 for each pregnancy, a value 25 times greater. Should we proscribe consanguineous marriages? In 16 states and the District of Columbia consanguinity laws are based on the Book of Leviticus in the Old Testament. Although first-cousin marriages are illegal in many states, the actual risk of first-cousin parents having a child with a recessive inherited disease is less than 1% according to a large and well-documented study. Accordingly, the risk for second cousins would be even lower. The danger of such unions is exaggerated in the public mind. Of course, the risk is entirely different for cousin marriages in pedigrees with known autosomal recessive disease.

Curt Stern has said, "The brotherhood of man is not only a spiritual concept but a genetic reality." Each person alive today had 2^{30} or approximately 10^9 ancestors 30 generations ago (750 to 1000 years ago). However, the population of the world at that time was less than 10^9, perhaps 10 times less, although exact estimates are unavailable. Thus

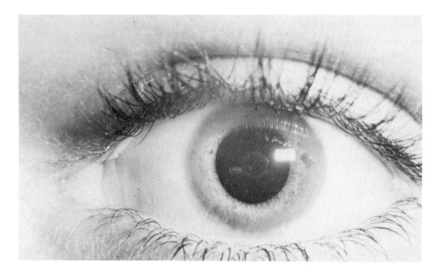

FIGURE 20. The painful fact about Wilson's disease is that its rarity impedes its recognition even when the physician is looking directly at the pathognomonic Kayser-Fleischer rings, missed by Wilson himself. Early intervention is essential.

we share our ancestors from a pool much smaller than the theoretical number that disregards consanguinity.

Because of the Hardy–Weinberg equilibrium, recessive genes are common in the general population. Normal persons are estimated to carry three to eight deleterious, recessive genes. When the diagnosis of an autosomal recessive disorder is made for a child, the parents may feel somehow guilty and abnormal for being carriers. We must remember that such parents differ from the rest of us only in the identification of one of their "bad" recessive genes and in the knowledge that they share this gene.

The abundance of heterozygotes relative to homozygotes for recessive diseases is related to the characteristic severity of recessive diseases: The total absence of genetic fitness, even the death of an afflicted homozygote, is of little consequence to the continued maintenance of a gene pool in society. Conversely, does treatment of genetic diseases perpetuate and increase the deleterious gene pool with consequent greater harm to future society? For the autosomal recessive diseases the effect of treatment on future generations is almost negligible: Remember that for every patient with Wilson's disease, treated and in candidacy for parenthood, there are 1000 unidentified carriers propagating the gene.

Survival and parenthood of patients with genetic disorders creates new problems for management of pregnancies. Thus the high concentrations of phenylalanine in a phenylketonuric mother will damage the developing brain of her infant in utero. The infant acquires damage from a genetic disease but by an environmental route. What is the effect of copper or of penicillamine on the unborn infant of a mother with Wilson's disease?

AUTOSOMAL DOMINANT INHERITANCE

Huntington's chorea, achondroplasia, tuberous sclerosis (Figure 21), and Marfan's syndrome are examples of about 1200 diseases so far known to be inherited in the autosomal dominant mode. The pedigrees (Figure 22) are characterized by affliction of both sexes, in the ratio of 1:1 with normal children, and with one affected parent. The appearance of the disorder in every generation of the pedigree gives a vertical pattern.

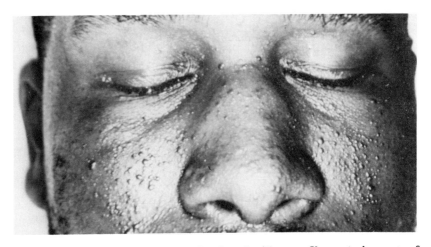

FIGURE 21. Tuberous sclerosis may be classed with neurofibromatosis as one of the hereditary neurocutaneous syndromes. The disorder is characterized by mental deficiency, convulsive seizures, and adenoma sebaceum, shown here. Actually the skin lesions are fibromas, not adenomas. Areas of malformed cerebral cortex, often calcified, comprise the brain lesions.

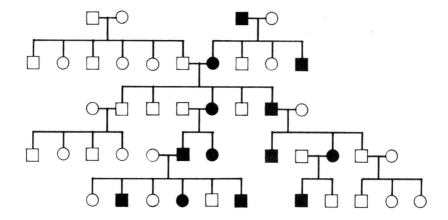

■● -Affected male, female   □○-Unaffected male, female

FIGURE 22. Idealized pedigree of an autosomal dominant trait. This pedigree does not reveal the tendency for most autosomal dominant diseases to be eliminated in a given pedigree.

One general characteristic of autosomal dominant disorders is marked variation in penetrance, or intensity of expression (Figure 23). In some cases a known gene carrier will have no manifestation of the disorder, and this phenomenon is called nonpenetrance. In fully penetrant dominant conditions the normal child of an affected parent will not have any affected progeny. Expression of a disorder can vary not only quantitatively but qualitatively. Thus a single gene defect is sometimes expressed in different ways in different organs or tissues with no obvious mechanism by which to connect the whole phenotype. Such pleiotropy is evident, for example, in Peutz-Jeghers syndrome (Figure 24), in which melanin spots on the digits, lips, and oral mucosa are somehow expressions of a defect also giving hamartomatous polyps in the small and large intestine.

Expression of a gene may differ in males and females. Thus baldness is autosomal dominant in males but autosomal recessive in females, who are bald only if homozygous for the baldness gene. Another example is the adrenogenital syndrome, caused by a defect in steroid 21-hydroxylase: In females virilization is ordinarily present at birth, whereas affected males are often not recognized until they manifest rapid growth in childhood or precocious puberty.

We should not expect to find defective enzymes as the basis for the disease in dominant disorders, because most reactions in living cells are substrate-limited, not enzyme-limited, and therefore, the halving of an enzyme concentration in a living cell should not be sufficient to give the disease phenotype. We have already seen that heterozygotes for most enzyme defects appear to be normal. Thus the dominant form of methemoglobinemia is caused by a defective hemoglobin whose presence as approximately half of the total hemoglobin causes the disease phenotype. By contrast, the recessive form of methemoglobinemia is caused by a defect in methemoglobin reductase, and activity must be well below half the normal level for the disease phenotype to result.

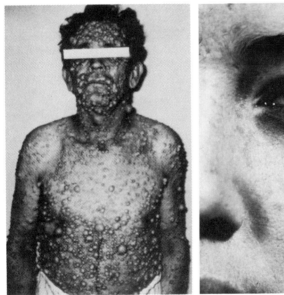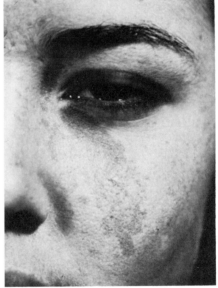

FIGURE 23. Marked variation of expression or penetrance is characteristic of autosomal dominant disorders. Here one patient with neurofibromatosis has hundreds of cutaneous tumors, whereas another has only multiple café-au-lait spots. Usually affected persons have more than six café-au-lait spots, and freckling in the axilla is characteristic. Even a mildly affected person is subject to later development of tumors in the central nervous system.

First patient from Dunn FG, DeCarvalho JGR, Kem DC, et al: Pheochromocytoma crisis induced by saralasin. N Engl J Med 295:605–607, 1976.

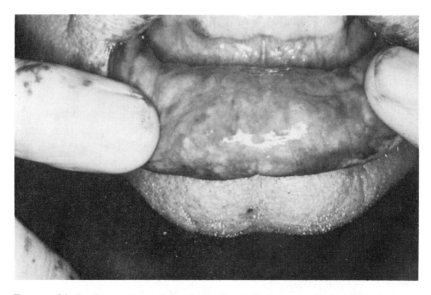

FIGURE 24. In the autosomal dominant Peutz-Jeghers syndrome melanin spots on the lips and digits signal hamartomatous polyps in the small and/or large intestine. Because of the Mendelian pattern of inheritance, a single defective gene must be responsible for the diverse phenotypic expression. This is an example of pleiotropy.

Familial hypercholesterolemia (Figure 25) is an autosomal dominant condition afflicting perhaps one of every 500 people. Here the defect is in a cell membrane protein which acts as a specific receptor for serum low-density lipoprotein, bearing cholesterol. In one form of the disorder, the receptors have a lowered binding affinity for cholesterol–low-density lipoprotein. In another form of the disorder, cells have only one half of the normal number of functioning receptors. The resultant decrease in absorptive-endocytosis diminishes the normal level of cholesterol released intracellularly for suppression of cholesterol synthesis and for stimulation of cholesterol esterification. Thus, serum cholesterol levels become set at about twice the normal level to reestablish control of cholesterol metabolism.

Most autosomal dominant diseases are not observed in the homozygous form, which is generally incompatible with life. Familial hypercholesterolemia is interesting in this respect, because the homozygous form is actually observable, although only at a frequency of about one in one million population. The gene dose effect is evident

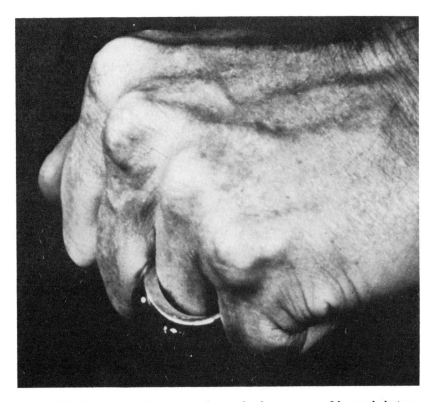

FIGURE 25. Tendon or tuberous xanthomas in the presence of hypercholestero-lemia and a family history of both make the diagnosis of familial hypercholes-terolemia. Xanthelasma and corneal arcus are often present but are less specific, sometimes occurring in the face of normal serum lipid levels.

in comparisons of the heterozygote and homozygote. Thus, the mean level of cholesterol–low-density lipoprotein in heterozygotes is double that of unaffected people of similar age, and the level in homozygotes is double that of heterozygotes. Heterozygotes have hypercholester-olemia from birth, develop coronary atherosclerosis and tendon xan-thomas in early adulthood, and have early myocardial infarction: one half of males by age 50. Homozygotes have severe hypercholestero-lemia from birth, develop generalized atherosclerosis in childhood, exhibit not only tendon xanthomas but yellow-orange cutaneous xan-thomas present by age 4, and die before 30 years of age from my-ocardial infarction.

For those diseases inherited in the dominant mode and evident at birth, the afflicted individuals are heterozygotes who immediately become subjected to natural selective forces and who for sociological and/or physiological reasons have a lowered reproductive rate, called lowered genetic fitness. There is no gene pool carried in unaffected people as there is for diseases of the recessive mode. Therefore, the severe diseases of the dominant mode of inheritance tend to be eliminated within a given pedigree, and such diseases continue to exist only by the occurrence of new mutations. For example, one study revealed the genetic fitness of achondroplasia to be 20%: Dwarfs had 20% of the number of children had by dwarf siblings. For this reason the majority of achondroplastic dwarfs are born to normal parents, one of whom has had a new mutation in a germ cell. Such parents would be no more likely than any other person to have another child with achondroplasia, a situation to be contrasted to the heterozygous parents of children with cystic fibrosis. Table 1 shows what percentage of patients with various dominant disorders represent fresh mutations.

TABLE 1
Fresh Mutation in Dominant Disorders

CONDITION	% FRESH MUTATION
Achondroplasia	80
Tuberous sclerosis	80
Neurofibromatosis	40
Marfan's syndrome	30
Myotonic dystrophy	25
Huntington's chorea	4
Adult polycystic kidney disease	1
Familial hypercholesterolemia	<1

From Goldstein JL, Brown MS: Genetic aspects of human disease, in Thorn GW, et al (eds): Harrison's Principles of Internal Medicine. New York, McGraw-Hill, 1977.

Of course, mild dominant disorders that do not measurably decrease genetic fitness persist in the population without dependence on fresh mutations. Although severe, Huntington's chorea is an exception of the tendency of diseases of dominant mode to die out in a given pedigree, because onset of this disease usually follows the reproductive period of life. Therefore, genetic fitness is not reduced sufficiently to eliminate the disorder. Most patients with this disease in the United

States are believed to have descended from one of three brothers. Acute intermittent porphyria is another exception. Another hepatic porphyria, the variegate porphyria common in South Africa, is present in at least 9000 people, all of whom are descendants of a single Dutch couple married in 1688. This is an example of the founder effect, whereby a gene has a particularly high frequency in a given population, because it is introduced by a founder who is a rare, nonrepresentative sample from a larger population.

Since affected persons constitute the major gene bank for the autosomal dominant diseases, successful treatment of those diseases will increase their incidences. For example, the completely successful treatment of the hereditary form of retinoblastoma, an autosomal dominant disease, would increase its incidence 100-fold in 2000 years.

MUTATION RATE

The mutation rates of various genes in man can be measured directly if the mutation produces a fully penetrant, dominant phenotype. In that case every affected child born to normal parents represents a fresh mutation. The mutation rate for achondroplasia calculated by this direct method is 4.2×10^{-5}. Dominant phenotypes are also useful in determination of mutation rates by the indirect method, which is based on the assumption that the disorder persists in the population in a steady state, new cases from fresh mutations being balanced by loss of mutants because of decreased genetic fitness. This equation can be expressed:

mutation rate = (selective disadvantage) (gene frequency)

for a given gene. Selective disadvantage is simply the decrease in genetic fitness. For achondroplasia we have already seen the selective disadvantage to be 80%. By use of the binomial expansion, $(p+q)^2 = p^2 + 2pq + q^2$, we can relate the gene frequencies of the normal (p) and achondroplasia (q) genes to the incidence of normals (p^2), heterozygotes ($2pq$), and homozygotes (q^2) in the population. In an actual population of 94,075 there were 10 achondroplastic dwarfs. Therefore, $2pq + q^2 = \dfrac{10}{94,075} = 1.06 \times 10^{-4}$. For a rare dominant trait homozygotes are negligible (or $q^2 \to 0$), and $p \simeq 1$. Therefore, as a close approximation $2q = 1.06 \times 10^{-4}$ and $q = 0.53 \times 10^{-4}$. Therefore the mutation rate $= (80\%)(0.53 \times 10^{-4}) = 4.2 \times 10^{-5}$. The equation is difficult to apply to autosomal recessive phenotypes, because of the preponderance of heterozygotes with indeterminate selective disadvantage (or advantage) over homozygotes.

For tuberous sclerosis the rate is approximately one mutation per 100,000 gametes. The lowest known rate in man, $1/10^6$, is that for

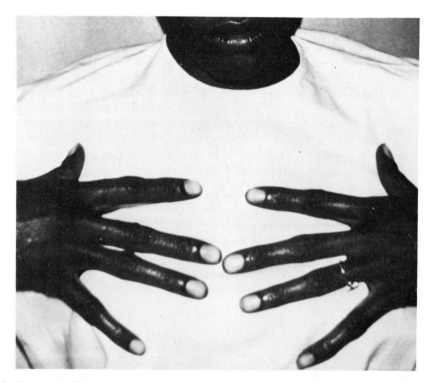

FIGURE 26. Marfan's syndrome is an autosomal dominant disorder characterized by long, thin toes and fingers (arachnodactyly), and dislocated lenses as shown at right. Patients may also have deformities of the thoracic cage, high arched palate, inguinal hernias, and unusually long extremities. Degenerative changes in the aortic media lead to dissecting aneurysm and rupture, and weakening of the aortic ring causes aortic regurgitation with congestive heart failure. Almost all deaths result from these cardiovascular complications.

Eye from Shih VE, Abroms IF, Johnson JL, et al: Sulfite oxidase deficiency: Investigations of a hereditary metabolic disorder. N Engl J Med 297:1022–1028, 1977.

Huntington's chorea. The highest known mutation rate in man is that for neurofibromatosis, $1/10^4$. These rates are comparable to mutation rates measured accurately in bacteria. For both Marfan's disease (Figure 26) and achondroplasia, the apparent mutation rate becomes greater for older fathers, and this is called the paternal age effect.

X-LINKED RECESSIVE INHERITANCE

The classical example of X-linked recessive inheritance is hemophilia or factor VIII deficiency. A fresh mutation in Queen Victoria or in the germ line of one of her parents made her the initial carrier in the British Royal Family. The mode of transmission was recognized by Talmudic

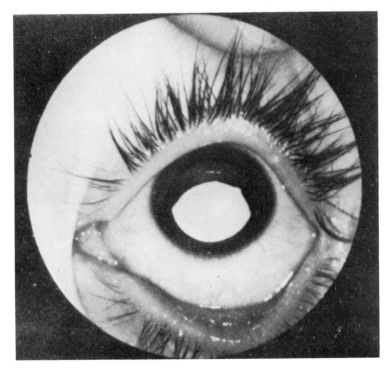

FIGURE 26. Continued.

laws regarding circumcision in the second century, AD, and was well described in the early 19th century before Gregor Mendel was born. However, the description remained a sterile empirical observation without the concepts of genes, chromosomes, and genetic ratios that appeared during the following 100 years.

The factor VIII gene is on the X chromosome, as are more than 100 other genes so far mapped. Without known exception these same genes reside on the X chromosome of all other mammals. Most of the X-linked disorders are inherited in the recessive mode, illustrated in Figure 27. There are no corresponding loci on the Y chromosome, so that males (XY) are hemizygous and carrying females (XX) are heterozygous for these recessive traits, of which red–green color blindness is another example.

The pedigree reveals that an affected male never transmits the disease to his son. However, all daughters of affected males are carriers. Half of the female carriers' sons are affected, and half of the female carriers' daughters are carriers. Affected (homozygous) women are

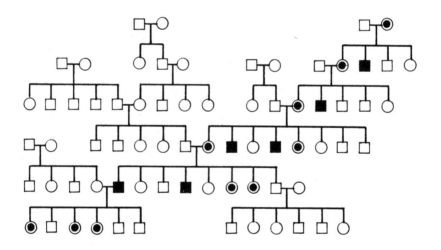

■-Affected males ◉-Carrier females □○-Unaffected males, females

FIGURE 27. Idealized pedigree of an X-linked recessive trait. Involvement of uncles and nephews gives an oblique pattern.

usually not seen, because they could arise only from the mating of an affected male with a carrier female. Females with XO Turner's syndrome are hemizygous and are affected in the same way males are affected by hemophilia and other X-linked recessive disorders.

The same risk of disease in male offspring is present for a carrier female regardless of her mate. Therefore, the notion that consanguinity is the basis for the prevalence of hemophilia in the British Royal Family is false.

The classical pedigree has an oblique character likened to the knight's move in chess, because of the involvement of uncles and nephews related through the female. For an X-linked recessive disorder with low fitness, perhaps one third of patients will have the classical pedigree. Another one third will be fresh mutations, and the remaining one third will be sons of fresh mutant carriers.

The Hardy–Weinberg law applies to X-linked loci, as well. Females, with two X chromosomes, exhibit the same genotype distribution observed for an autosomal locus: $p^2 + 2pq + q^2$. However, males, with only one X chromosome, directly reflect the gene frequencies in the ratio of normal (p) to hemophilia (q) phenotypes, with no heterozygotes. Therefore, the incidence of affected females (q^2) is the square of the incidence of affected males (q). Consequently, the more rare the disease in males, the greater will be the discrepancy in incidence between males and females: if one male in 100 shows the trait, the expected female frequency will be 100-fold lower; if one male in 1000 shows the trait, the expected female frequency will be 1000-fold lower.

Glucose-6-phosphate dehydrogenase (G6PD) deficiencies affect 100 million males worldwide, comprise the most common X-linked disorder and the most common enzyme deficiency in man. More than 100 variants are described, some causing no clinical manifestations. The African, Mediterranean, and Canton types occur most often. Because 12% of American black males have the disorder, about 21% of American black females are carriers. An expected 1.4% of black females are homozygous for the trait, being progeny of affected males and carrier females. The G6PD deficiency is important in ecogenetics as an example of a genetic abnormality elicited by environmental factors including foods and drugs harmless to the rest of the population.

In X-linked recessive traits without known enzyme defects to assay, female relatives of affected males may seek premarital genetic counseling. In the pedigree shown in Figure 28, Mary's grandmother must be a carrier, because she has two affected sons. Although Jane had a 0.5 probability of being a carrier before her marriage, that chance is substantially decreased by her having mothered two normal sons. The joint probability of being a carrier and having two normal sons is (0.5) (0.25) = 0.125, and the joint probability of *not* being a carrier and having two normal sons is (0.5) (1.0) = 0.5. Therefore, the probability that Jane is *not* a carrier is four times the probability that Jane *is* a carrier. Because Jane must either *be* or *not be* a carrier, the probability that she is a carrier is 0.2. Therefore, Mary's initial probability of being a carrier is only 0.1 before her marriage. Each normal son Mary bears will in turn decrease her probability of being a carrier.

Because of the Lyon phenomenon, females heterozygous for X-linked traits vary from no expression to full expression of the trait. Therefore, enzyme assays may not reliably detect certain carriers whereas other carriers may exhibit the disease phenotype. Consider

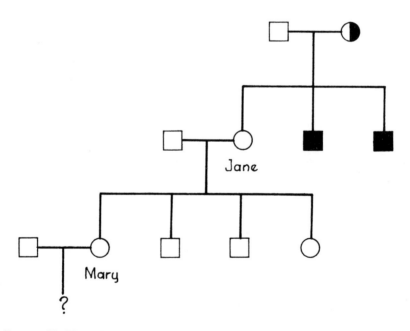

FIGURE 28. The existence of Mary's two normal brothers decreases the probabilities that Jane and Mary are carriers for hemophilia.

the pedigree in Figure 29. The father had clinical hemophilia. All three daughters were thus obligatory carriers. One daughter had no measurable factor VIII and had clinical hemophilia. The second daughter had 50% of normal factor VIII levels and was clinically normal. The third daughter had normal factor VIII levels but bore a son with clinical hemophilia, thereby proving her carrier status. In genetic counseling for X-linked recessive diseases all potential carriers should be identified not only out of concern for their progeny but because preventive measures may prevent expression of the disease in the carrier herself.

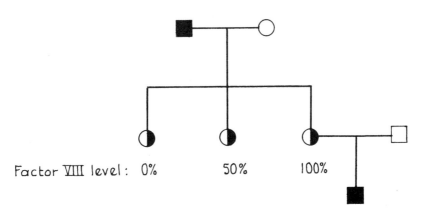

Factor VIII level: 0%   50%   100%

FIGURE 29. The finding of normal factor VIII activity does not exclude the possibility of one's being a hemophilia carrier.

X-LINKED DOMINANT INHERITANCE

In X-linked dominant disorders, both males and females are affected (although females are affected twice as often as males), and both transmit the disorder to their children. The pedigree pattern is vertical and resembles that of the autosomal dominant disorders except that the affected father transmits the disease to *none* of his sons and to *all* of his daughters, whereas the affected mother transmits to one half of her sons and to one half of her daughters. Because of the random inactivation of one X chromosome early in female embryogenesis (Lyon phenomenon), X-linked dominant disorders tend to be less severe in females than in males. All of these criteria are met by hereditary nephritis as defined by hematuria in two large pedigrees. Another X-linked dominant disorder is pseudohypoparathyroidism. This disorder is the result of defective response of target cells to parathormone. [Other genetic disorders of defective target cell response to hormones are nephrogenic diabetes insipidus (ADH) and testicular feminization (androgens), both X-linked].

DEFINITION OF PHENOTYPE MAY DETERMINE
MODE OF INHERITANCE

The usefulness of the concepts of dominance and recessiveness may turn to confusion in situations with codominant alleles, as those for the normal hemoglobin β chain and the sickle cell β chain. Here one must realize that phenotype may be redefined for different levels of observation. If the phenotype is defined as sickle cell disease with its usual clinical manifestations, then the mode of inheritance is autosomal recessive. However, if the phenotype is defined as the in vitro sickling (Figure 30) phenomenon, then the mode of inheritance is autosomal dominant. An understanding of how a definition of phenotype determines dominance or recessiveness helps in the sometimes frustrating attempt to keep pace with and to comprehend current literature. In 1977 three articles on familial hemochromatosis appeared in the New England Journal of Medicine. For this disease the hereditary nature and the mode of inheritance have been debated for years. In one sense these three articles compounded the confusion, because two supported an autosomal dominant mode and one supported an autosomal recessive mode of inheritance. The explanation for this apparent disagreement reveals that no disagreement really exists, because the writers have chosen two different definitions of hemochromatosis. The article supporting a recessive mode defined hemochromatosis as the presence of melanoderma and hepatomegaly in the face of demonstrated iron overload, with serum iron and unsaturated iron-binding capacity and desferrioxamine test being abnormal in all cases. Some patients had diabetes mellitus, some had hypogonadism, some cardiac abnormalities, and some arthropathy. The articles supporting a dominant mode emphasized that the earliest change in the disease is abnormal hepatic iron level, and they defined that change as early hemochromatosis if

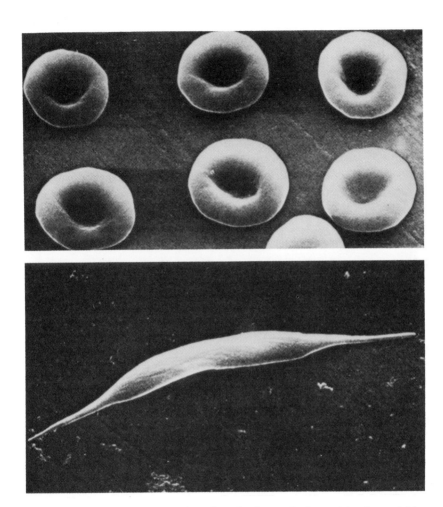

FIGURE 30. The red blood cell is unique in that a single protein, hemoglobin, comprises 34% of the cell (mean corpuscular hemoglobin concentration). Consequently, the polymerization of sickle hemoglobin is an event that physically alters the entire red blood cell. The rigid, sickled cells obstruct capillary blood flow and ultimately lead to the clinical vaso-occlusive crises characteristic of sickle-cell anemia. In sickle-cell trait, vaso-occlusive crises do not occur under normal conditions, because the concentration of sickle hemoglobin is insufficient.

From Sickle cell anemia faces new attack. Chem. Eng. News Jan 6:16–17, 1975.

other family members were affected. None of their patients had melanoderma and hepatomegaly and the other late changes, and even
serum iron, unsaturated iron-binding capacity, and desferrioxamine
tests were normal in many affected patients. Thus by the most sensi-
tive test, hepatic iron level, the heterozygotes are detectable, a dominant situation, whereas the overt disease appears in homozygotes and
is therefore recessive. Other factors such as age, alcohol consumption,
and sex (pregnancies and menstrual blood loss) are important modi-
fiers, and the possibility that certain heterozygotes will develop the
full disease remains likely but unproven. Until we become able to
identify the genotype in patients with familial hemochromatosis, one
genetic model is consistent with all the data available so far: the disease
is Mendelian and appears in all homozygotes for the hemochromatosis
gene on chromosome 6. Heterozygotes have increased iron stores in
the liver by middle adulthood and may go on to develop overt disease
in the face of increased alcohol consumption or may be protected from
overt disease by iron loss via menses, pregnancy, or phlebotomy. I
shall discuss the role of exogenous and environmental factors in
expression of genetic disease more fully in a later chapter.

We must avoid the impression that patients with genetic disorders
always present a positive pedigree. Often the reverse is true, and no
pedigree analysis is possible, as shown in Figure 31. This situation is
understandable in light of the phenomenon of fresh mutations and in
view of the smaller size of modern families. Thus more than one half
(9/16) of two-children families with both parents carrying the same
autosomal recessive trait will have no affected children, and only 1/16
of such families will have two affected children.

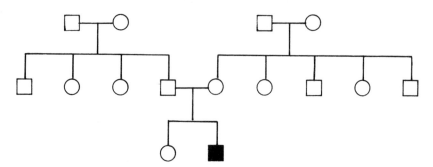

FIGURE 31. Patients with chromosomal, Mendelian, or polygenic disorders frequently present an otherwise negative pedigree.

LEGAL GENETICS

Paternity testing is a genetic–legal interface arising directly from Mendelian genetics. The factors studied must be inherited in a Mendelian pattern, present at birth, and stable throughout life. Systems in use are erythrocyte and leukocyte antigens, serum proteins, erythrocyte enzymes, and HLA typing. By use of 24 such systems, a 99% chance exists to exclude a putative but not actual father, but a putative father cannot be proved to be the actual father.

The obligation of physicians to recognize Mendelian disorders and to inform relatives at risk is another question with legal implications. The problem is particularly pertinent when the disorder is insidious in onset and is affected by environmental factors or is preventable or treatable. Examples are hemochromatosis, porphyria cutanea tarda, Wilson's disease, and multiple endocrine adenomatosis.

ASSOCIATION OF GENETIC
MARKERS AND DISEASES

Certain diseases of unknown cause occur in association with markers identifiable biochemically or immunologically and inherited in an identifiable Mendelian manner, even though the role (if any) of the marker in pathogenesis is obscure. Such diseases may demonstrate family clustering but seldom a clearcut Mendelian pattern of inheritance. I shall consider these associations now. They illustrate genetic principles that are useful in the understanding and management of diseases such as ankylosing spondylitis.

Recently, enormous attention has focused on the association of certain histocompatibility antigens with specific diseases. Whereas the ABO blood group antigens are the major determinants of red blood cell compatibility, the major barriers to transplantation of nucleated cells in man are the HLAs (for human leukocyte antigens), which penetrate the plasma membranes of all nucleated cells (Figure 32). The HLA system is unique among systems of genetic markers by its association with a wide variety of diseases.

Pregnant women are frequently immunized against paternally derived fetal HLAs, probably because fetal lymphocytes pass into the maternal circulation. However, feto–maternal HLA incompatibility is of no clinical significance. Sera of multiparous women are sources for the antibodies used to type the HLAs. The test measures killing, in the presence of complement, of donor lymphocytes by sera containing antibodies to the lymphocyte HLAs.

The major histocompatibility complex (MHC) is on the short arm of chromosome 6 and includes the HLA loci as well as loci for complements $C2$ and $C4$. The four loci, HLA–A, HLA–B, HLA–C, and HLA–D, are closely linked and highly polymorphic. In fact, the polymorphism of these loci exceeds that of any other known genetic sys-

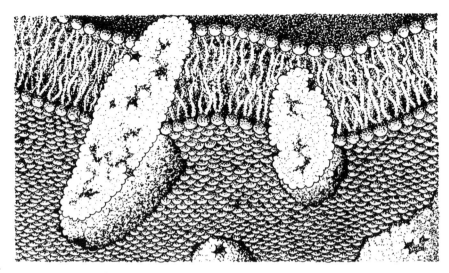

FIGURE 32. Cell membrane. The HLA antigens are glycoproteins extending through the lipid bilayer as schematized here.

Adapted from a drawing by B Tagawa from Singer SJ: Architecture and topography of biologic membranes. Hospital Practice 8(5) 1973; and from Weissman G, Claiborne R (eds): Cell Membranes: Biochemistry, Cell Biology, and Pathology. New York, HP Publishing Co., 1975.

tem, with the special exception of the immunoglobulin variable region. For n possible alleles at a single locus, there are $n(n + 1)/2$ possible genotypes. Thus, 22 alleles at the HLA–B locus would give $22 \cdot 23/2 = 253$ possible genotypes. When this number is combined with similar figures calculated for the other loci, an enormous variability in genotypes for the four loci is available. Most of the HLAs so far designated and used in clinical testing and literature are alleles at the A and B loci.

A haplotype consists of the genes in a region of one of the chromosomes of a pair. The haplotypes on the two chromosomes of the pair make up the genotype. Each person carries two HLA haplotypes, one on the maternally derived and one on the paternally derived chromosome 6. For example, a genotype for the A and B loci might be $\dfrac{A3\ B8}{A11\ B7}$, with one haplotype written above and one below the line.

Since the number of alleles is large, the likelihood that two unrelated people would have the same four alleles at HLA–A and B is very low. Each child of a given couple shares one haplotype with each parent, but he could not be identical to the parent in HLA genotype unless the parents had one haplotype in common. This is the basis for difficulty in matching parents and children for renal transplantation. However, two siblings have one chance in four of being HLA identical (on the assumption that no crossovers occur), and consequently siblings are the more likely source for organ transplants.

The HLAs A, B, and C are glycoproteins of 45,000 in molecular weight, closely associated with β_2 microglobulin, a protein of 12,000 in molecular weight. The β_2 microglobulin is synthesized by nearly every cell in the body, is invariant in structure within a species, and carries none of the antigenic determinants of the HLAs. Human β_2 microglobulin has been completely sequenced and is homologous to the constant domains of immunoglobulin light and heavy chains, a fact suggesting a common ancestral gene. The gene for β_2 microglobulin is on chromosome 15, thus completely independent of the MHC.

The products of genes in the D region are involved in and designated by the mixed-lymphocyte-culture test, in which lymphocytes of unlike HLA–D antigens undergo blastogenesis when placed together in tissue culture. The D region is comparable to the murine I region, which contains the immune response genes that determine whether a certain antigen will provoke an immune response. The HLA-D antigens may be the B lymphocyte alloantigens, which consist of a protein of 33,000 in molecular weight specified by the D locus and of a protein of 25,000 in molecular weight specified by another chromosome.

One of the earliest and strongest associations of idiopathic disease with an HLA antigen was the relation of ankylosing spondylitis (Figure 33) to HLA–B27. The data can be expressed in a hypothetical two-by-two contingency table for 100,000 white Americans:

Ankylosing spondylitis	HLA–B27		
	+	−	Total
+	1,400	74	1,474
−	5,600	92,926	98,526
Total	7,000	93,000	100,000

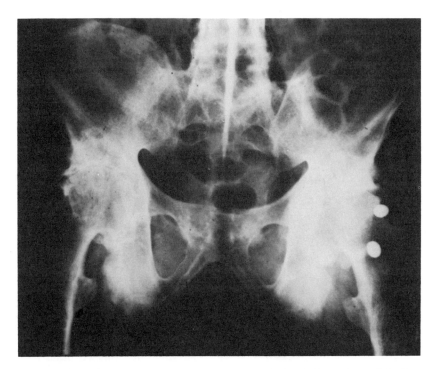

FIGURE 33. Ankylosing spondylitis is easily recognized when the radiological features are fully developed. These include ossification of the annulus fibrosus of the intervertebral discs, fusion of the sacroiliac joints, fusion of the symphysis pubis, syndesmophytes bridging adjacent vertebrae, both rarefaction and new bone formation in the pelvis, and involvement of the hips.

The table shows that HLA–B27 is present in 95% of 1,474 patients with ankylosing spondylitis. In the total group of 100,000, 7% have antigen, and of those 7%, 20% develop the disease. In contrast, the risk of developing the disease is only about 0.08% (74 of 93,000 people) among those negative for B27. Therefore, a person with the B27 antigen is 250 times more likely to develop ankylosing spondylitis than a person lacking that antigen. Other studies have placed this relative risk closer to 100, but the helpfulness of B27 determination in diagnosis remains.

Such associations have been reported for nearly 50 diseases, and while viewing the data with skepticism until confirmation arrives, we can form a mental framework for this information by an explanation of what such associations mean.

One explanation for such observations is a sampling artifact called ethnic stratification. Here both the disease and the designated antigen exist in higher frequencies in a subpopulation drawn from a heterogeneous population, but the antigen bears no causal relationship to the disease, and the genes for each are not linked. A second explanation for an observed association is that the antigen is causally connected to the disease. The role of the antigen could be direct or indirect. If causation were the explanation for an observed association, then the specified HLA would be required for the disease state, and at least some other alleles would never be associated with the disease. In no such case has such a mechanism yet been described, but causation in pathogenesis seems plausible, both because other loci concerned with the immune system are closely linked to the HLA complex on chromosome 6, and because in the mouse, certain histocompatibility antigens alter immunological responses and susceptibility to viral infections.

A third explanation for an observed association is linkage disequilibrium. Linkage disequilibrium is the occurrence of two alleles at linked loci in haplotype frequencies greater than expected from the product of their individual frequencies—that expected by chance. Linkage disequilibrium is a striking characteristic of the HLA system. For example, in caucasians, HLA–A1 and HLA–B8 have gene frequencies of 0.14 and 0.10, respectively, and should occur together in 0.014 of haplotypes. In fact, however, the haplotype frequency of HLA–A1, HLA–B8 in caucasians is 0.064, a significantly greater number. The basis for the many linkage disequilibria in the HLA system is not understood. At present, the best way to explain both the linkage disequilibrium and the extreme polymorphism of the HLA system is to ascribe these characteristics of the system to selective forces and events in evolution. Nevertheless, a gene, or genes, responsible for a disease associated with a specific HLA may be linked to the MHC and in linkage disequilibrium with the allele for the HLA.

Family studies, in contrast to population studies, provide evidence for linkage of certain disease loci with the HLA loci, even when no *particular* HLA allele is associated with the disease in the population at large. As explained earlier, linkage refers to the physical connection of two or more gene loci. Genes on the same chromosome are physically linked and remain so unless crossing over occurs in meiosis. When gene loci are transmitted to the same gamete with a frequency higher than the 50% expectation of Mendel's law of independent assortment, they are linked. When a disease gene locus is linked to the HLA complex, then the occurrence of a given HLA haplotype in a family with the disease can serve as a marker for the disease gene. More importantly, the given HLA haplotype can serve as a predictor of the disease and can allow prophylactic surveillance or improved counseling or both. Examples from the recent literature include spinocerebellar ataxia, hemochromatosis, and juvenile diabetes mellitus.

One form of spinocerebellar ataxia is determined by an allele at a locus linked to the HLA locus on chromosome 6. A study of the HLA haplotypes and the disease in a large pedigree revealed that the apparent connection is 1400 times more likely to exist because of linkage than because of chance (lod score of 3.15 for a recombination fraction of 0.12). The linkage distance of 12 cM predicts that recombinants (from crossing over) will exist in only 12% of gametes. Therefore, prediction of disease development based on the HLA typing of a child in this family is 88% accurate. Because the disease is autosomal dominant with late onset (at 20 to 40 years of age), counseling without the HLA typing is confined to prediction that a child of an affected person has a 50% chance of becoming affected. Such counseling is all that is now available in Huntington's chorea, for example. Thus linkage studies enormously refine predictive accuracy and resultant counseling.

In the case of hemochromatosis, both population and family studies have illuminated the genetic basis for the disease. Population studies have revealed strong association of HLA-A3 ($P < 10^{-11}$) and HLA-B14 ($P < 10^{-8}$) with the overt disease. However, neither of these antigens is necessary or present in all cases. Therefore, causation can be ruled out as the basis for the association, and linkage disequilibrium would appear to be the explanation. Family studies confirm the linkage of the hemochromatosis gene to the HLA complex on chromosome 6 with a Lod score of 2.239 for a recombination fraction of 0.005 (odds 173 to 1 for linkage so tight that cross overs only exist in 0.5% of the gametes). Moreover, family studies show that affected siblings ordinarily have identical HLA genotypes ($P < 10^{-4}$). Therefore, such persons have inherited HLA-hemochromatosis haplotypes from each parent, and the overt form of the disease is autosomal recessive. A practical consequence of this study is the ability provided to predict with high accuracy the development or nondevelopment of the disease among family members according to HLA genotype. Consequent corrective steps to alter the environmental risk factors can then be used. Those found to be heterozygous would be particularly advised to avoid alcohol, for example.

In juvenile diabetes mellitus the situation is more complicated, because of a penetrance factor. Identical twins have 50% concordance for juvenile diabetes mellitus, a figure that, if correct, indicates 50% penetrance. Now HLA studies reveal that siblings of index cases of juvenile diabetes mellitus have a 50% concordance if they are HLA identical but only a 6% concordance if not HLA identical, as shown in the two-by-two contingency table. The difference is highly significant ($P \simeq 0.0014$), and the HLA identity is evidence for an autosomal recessive mode of inheritance, because certain haplotypes seem to be required from each parent.

HLA	Diabetic	Nondiabetic	Total
Identical	6	6	12
Nonidentical	3	46	49
Total	9	52	61

However, the incomplete penetrance allows other explanations for the mode of inheritance. Nevertheless, siblings HLA identical to index cases of juvenile diabetes mellitus would appear to share the same risk for development of the disease (50%) as that of identical twins. The role of viral infections in juvenile diabetes mellitus opens interesting questions regarding the linkage to the HLA complex and again introduces the concept of environmental–genetic interactions to be discussed in the next chapter.

POLYGENIC OR
MULTIFACTORIAL
INHERITANCE

In our concentration on Mendelian traits and diseases determined by single genes, we must not overlook polygenic or multifactorial inheritance, for example, the inheritance of stature or of intelligence. Both exhibit the hallmark of a multifactorial phenotype: a continuous range of values expressed by a distribution curve, that is, continuous variation as distinct from the discontinuous variation of Mendelian phenotypes.

Congenital defects attributed to multifactorial inheritance include cleft lip and palate, dislocation of the hip, club foot, pyloric stenosis, hypospadias, atrial septal defect, patent ductus arteriosus, and tetralogy of Fallot. The actual recurrence rates among siblings and offspring of persons with these disorders ranges from 2 to 7%, numbers clearly not reflecting Mendelian ratios. Counseling must be based on empirical data.

What is the risk of having a baby with cleft palate if one's brother or aunt had cleft palate? The risk to family members is determined by degree of relatedness to an affected member. First-, second-, and third-degree relatives share one half, one fourth, and one eighth of their genes, respectively, with the designated person. First-degree relatives are one's parents, children, and siblings. The risk to relatives can be illustrated by a mathematical model, as shown in Figure 34. Imagine that ten gene loci strongly affect the appearance or nonappearance of a disorder, each risk allele n increasing and each nonrisk allele m decreasing the likelihood of the disorder. If m and n were equally distributed in the population, then the population could be represented by a symmetrical binomial distribution $(m+n)^{10}$ where $m = n = 5$, with

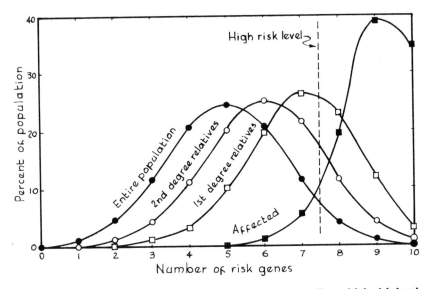

FIGURE 34. For polygenic disorders the probability of exceeding a high-risk level of inheritance is determined by the degree of genetic relation to an affected person.

an average of five risk alleles per individual. About 5% of people then have more than seven risk alleles and are in the high-risk zone for developing the disorder. In the model, most affected people have nine risk alleles and are represented by a skewed binomial distribution $(m+n)^{10}$ where $m = 1$ and $n = 9$. Since affected people comprise only 5% of the entire population, the distribution of unaffected people is almost identical to that drawn for the entire population with an average of five risk alleles.

Since a first-degree relative of an affected person shares an average of one half of genes with that person, most first-degree relatives have seven risk alleles (the average of five and nine) as shown by the skewed binomial distribution. When compared to the entire population, a higher percentage of people in this group exceed the high-risk threshold. In the same way, most second-degree relatives have six risk alleles. This group has more individuals above the high-risk level than the population at large, but not as many as the first-degree relatives. Third-degree relatives have an almost negligible added risk.

A notable and general feature of polygenic disorders is that the risk to relatives increases with the severity of the index case. This observation is not true of Mendelian disorders. Moreover, the striking variability of expression of autosomal dominant disorders provides no basis for prediction of severity. Thus a person mildly affected by neurofibromatosis cannot be assured that his affected children will also be only mildly affected.

ENVIRONMENTAL FACTORS

We call a disease "genetic" when its genetic causation overwhelms environmental factors. However, virtually all human diseases have genetic factors, and many reveal clear interactions of defined genetic and environmental elements. Thus porphyria cutanea tarda (PCT) was once believed to be an acquired disease, seen especially in alcoholics with hepatic siderosis. However, the vast majority of alcoholics with liver disease do not develop the bullous, photosensitive dermatitis characteristic of PCT (Figure 35). Those with PCT have a decrease in uroporphyrinogen decarboxylase, inherited in the autosomal dominant mode.

Genetic and environmental factors both play roles in such conditions as hypertension and adult onset diabetes mellitus. Even in "purely genetic" diseases, the environment is important in terms both of the total genetic constitution of the individual and in terms of exogenous factors, for example, administration of succinyl choline in pseudocholinesterase deficiency.

Congenital dislocation of the hip is perhaps the best studied of disorders resulting from convergence of hereditary and environmental factors. The genetic factors include familial joint laxity, which in mild form exists in 6% of normal school children, and acetabular dysgenesis, which is itself probably polygenic, because the depth of the acetabulum follows a normal distribution. The environmental factors include breech positioning in utero and the "swaddling factor," that is the position of the infant's lower extremities after birth: extended and adducted as in the papoose or flexed and abducted as in babies of Chinese peasants. (This latter position is produced by application of double diapers, used for therapy in this condition.) Furthermore, the

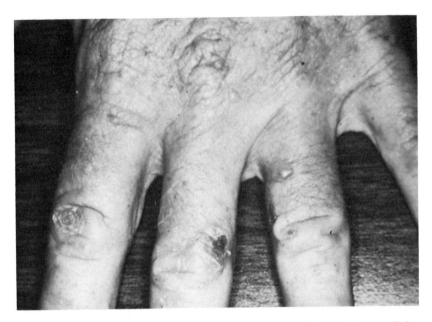

FIGURE 35. Perhaps 2% of chronic alcoholics develop vesicles or ulcers on light-exposed skin after minimal thermal or mechanical trauma as shown here by the small lesions on the fingers. The diagnosis of porphyria cutanea tarda can then be confirmed by demonstration of increased urinary porphyrin excretion. Acidified urine fluoresces red or pink. Two pathogenetic factors are important, one genetic, one environmental. The genetic factor is decreased uroporphyrinogen decarboxylase, an enzyme required for the biosynthesis of heme. The environmental factor is liver and total body iron overload. Treatment by phlebotomy to remove iron reverts urinary porphyrin excretion to normal, and skin sensitivity disappears, but enzyme levels remain unchanged. The mechanism by which alcohol aggravates or precipitates the disease remains unclear.

fivefold greater incidence in girls relative to boys may (speculatively) be explained by a temporary, relaxin-induced joint laxity in fetal and neonatal females. Eventually such an analysis may be possible for schizophrenia, which gives concordance of 45% in monozygotic twins, 10% in first-degree relatives, and 2% in second-degree relatives.

The interaction of heredity and environment varies with time and place. For example, the sickle cell trait and the G6PD defects, considered harmful in our environment, are positive factors for survival in areas of Africa where malaria is the leading cause of death. These are balanced polymorphisms; that is, significant fractions of the general population carry the variant gene, because the heterozygote is more fit than either homozygote.

Whereas sickle trait and G6PD deficiency provide partial protection against malaria, absolute protection, at least against *Plasmodium vivax*, is provided by the absence of the Duffy blood-group substance, which is apparently the cell membrane receptor necessary for penetration of the erythrocyte by the organism.

TWINS

The area of polygenic and multifactorial disease, because frequencies fail to follow the regularities of Mendelian predictions, has kept alive the use of twin studies in spite of inherent pitfalls. The idea is to distinguish between genetic and environmental factors by comparisons of concordance in monozygotic and dizygotic twins. Sometimes these twins are called "identical" and "nonidentical," but "identical" twins may not really be so. For example, monozygotic twins may exhibit different karyotypes and associated phenotypes, such as Down's syndrome and normal, because nondisjunction can occur in one and not in the other. Pairs of monozygotic twins of different sex have even been described (XY and XO). These examples are unusual. However, differential patterns of Lyonization of the X chromosomes in monozygotic female twins should commonly produce different phenotypic expression of associated traits. Most importantly, different environmental factors beginning even in the womb assure developmental differences in monozygotic twins.

Zygosity is determined by placentation or by similarity studies. Placentation can be unreliable, because monozygotic twins may have separate placentas, and conversely, dizygotic twins, although implanting separately, may fuse placentas to form a single organ difficult to distinguish grossly at the time of birth from a single placenta. Similarities of sex and of blood factors and HLA antigens can be used as in paternity testing to establish likelihood of mono- or dizygosity. Dermatoglyphic patterns may differ appreciably in monozygous twins, but when such patterns are identical, monozygosity is certain. The most dependable method for determination of zygosity is skin grafting.

Twin-birth frequency itself is influenced by both genetic and environmental factors. The frequency of monozygous twins is rather constant in all populations at three or four per 1000 births. However, dizygous twin frequencies vary markedly (by a factor of 17) as a function of the mother's race, but not the father's race. Dizygous twin frequencies are typically 20 per 1000 births for black Africans, six to ten per 1000 births for Europeans and caucasian Americans, and less than three per 1000 births for Japanese. Moreover, both maternal age and, independently, parity increase the frequency of dizygotic twin births. Familial factors are well known. Thus the sister of a woman with dizygous twins has double the normal probability of giving birth to dizygous twins. Socioeconomic factors have been shown to influence dizygous twinning frequencies in diverse populations.

HETEROGENEITY AND PHENOCOPIES

Linkage studies may permit distinction between identical phenotypes resulting from different genotypes. Thus two types of elliptocytosis are each autosomal dominant, but one is linked to the Rh blood group (chromosome 1), and the other is not so linked. Just as ancient physicians spoke of "the fever," we sometimes identify by a single name a disease actually caused by diverse and unrelated mutations, inherited in different ways. The phenomenon of identical phenotypes from diverse genotypes is called genetic heterogeneity (Figure 36). The examples of elliptocytosis and methemoglobinemia have been given. Another example is gout: one form results from overactive PRPP synthetase, inherited in an autosomal dominant mode, and another form results from deficient hypoxanthine-guanine phosphoribosyl transferase (HGPRTase), inherited in an X-linked recessive mode. Diabetes mellitus is certainly many different diseases. First, adult and juvenile types are clearly distinguishable clinically. Concordance for monozygotic twins is 100% for the adult type but only 50% for the juvenile type. The juvenile type can be clearly divided into a subtype that may be recessive and 50% penetrant with its gene linked to the HLA complex on chromosome 6 and an unusual subtype inherited in an autosomal dominant pattern. This form appears in childhood but lacks the severity of common juvenile diabetes mellitus and does not lead to vascular pathology.

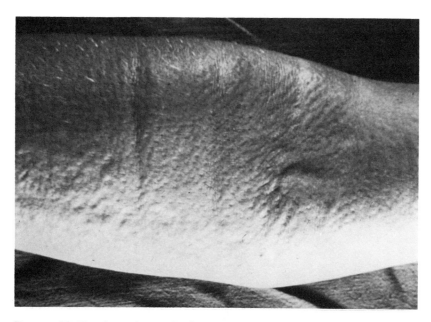

FIGURE 36. Pseudoxanthoma elasticum is a clinical syndrome with both auto-somal recessive and autosomal dominant forms, exemplifying genetic heteroge-neity. The basic defect, not understood at the biochemical level, becomes manifest histologically in altered elastic fibers, particularly in skin and in medium and small arteries. Resultant thick, loose, grooved skin occurs in areas such as the antecubital fossa shown here but including those not exposed to the sun, such as axillary and inguinal regions. Arterial changes lead to occlusion and to hemor-rhage. Patients typically present in the second to fourth decades of life with angina pectoris, intermittent claudication, hypertension, and recurrent gastroin-testinal bleeding. Angioid streaks are visible by routine retinoscopy.

These considerations are important in practice. Thus your adult pa-tient with a repaired cleft lip and palate may inquire about the risk to his or her children. Your reply cannot be casual or hasty. You must first determine, if possible, whether the defect occurred on a polygenic basis (most common), or on a single-gene basis (autosomal dominant when accompanied by lower lip pitting) or on a nongenetic basis (use of a drug such as diphenylhydantoin during pregnancy). Recall familial hypercholesterolemia, which constitutes less than 5% of cases of hy-percholesterolemia. Defects resembling genetic disorders but nonge-netic in origin are called phenocopies. These same questions can be raised regarding congenital heart disease. The counseling given will differ enormously for the various causations.

One should here review and confirm understanding of the terms congenital, familial, inherited, and genetic, often misapplied. Cleft palate is congenital but only partially inherited. Tuberculosis is not inherited but may be familial by contact, and genetic factors contribute to its natural history, different racial groups varying enormously in resistance to progression of the disease. Not only does increased concordance exist for tuberculosis in monozygotic twins, but the organ distribution and even the areas affected in the lungs are more uniform in monozygotic twins than in dizygotic twins.

BIOCHEMISTRY OF GENETIC EXPRESSION

Thy codons are as poetry
As writ by greatest Pen
In base sequential mysteries
Which chromatins defend.
Two sugar phosphate helices
Pyrimidines between
With purines neatly organized
Enumerate each gene...

Barbara S. Giesser, 1976

GENES ARE MADE OF DNA

In order to understand the mechanisms by which mutant genes produce disease, we must first understand the biochemistry of the genetic material and protein synthesis. Genes are made of DNA, a linear polymer of deoxyribonucleotidyl residues. All DNA in mammalian chromosomes consists of two such linear polymers aligned in antiparallel (defined below) fashion, hydrogen-bonded one to another according to the rules of specific purine-pyrimidine base pairing (Figure 37), and entwined in the double helical form first proposed by Watson and Crick (Figure 38). At any locus the genetic information in DNA is specified by the linear sequence of purine and pyrimidine bases in one of the two strands, the other strand serving as complementary "back up" information so that any repair necessary for the "sense" strand will be correct. In the process of cell division, the DNA content of the mother cell is exactly duplicated with separation of the two strands of the double helix and precise synthesis of new complementary strands, again according to the rules of base pairing. In this way genetic information is preserved without error from generation to generation. This process of replication is mediated by a complex of about ten enzymatic and structural proteins even in *Escherichia coli*, whose chromosome serves as a simple model for higher forms. The proteins have functions such as unwinding the DNA double helix, polymerizing new DNA

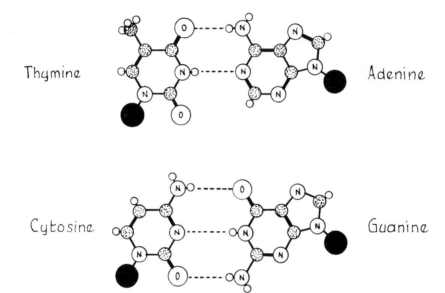

Thymine   Adenine

Cytosine   Guanine

FIGURE 37. Specific base pairing in DNA. The planar purine–pyrimidine base pairs form as shown in these ball-and-stick models. Hydrogen bonds are depicted by broken lines. Small circles are hydrogen atoms, and stippled circles are car-bom atoms. Oxygen and nitrogen atoms are labeled. The black circles are the carbon-1 atoms of deoxyribose, and are 11 Å apart in both base pairs. Thus, in the DNA double helix, adenine always pairs with thymine, and guanine always pairs with cytosine. In RNA, uracil replaces thymine to form the classical base pair with adenine. In the DNA double helix such base pairs are stacked on others to form a column in the center of the molecule with ten base pairs for each 360° turn of the phosphate–sugar "backbone."

from deoxynucleoside triphosphate precursors, and joining shorter segments to form the complete strand. Such strands extend the full length of human chromosomes, 48 to 240 million base pairs per chromosome.

DNA is the ultimate in miniaturization of information storage. All of the genetic information required to specify a human being is contained in about 6×10^{-12} gram of DNA (Figure 39). Even that amount is 50 to 100 times more than is needed to contain the estimated 50,000 genes coding for enzymatic and structural proteins. (For comparison E. coli has about 4,000 such genes, and the fruit fly has about 5,000.) The function of the remaining DNA is unknown, but much of it must be involved in control.

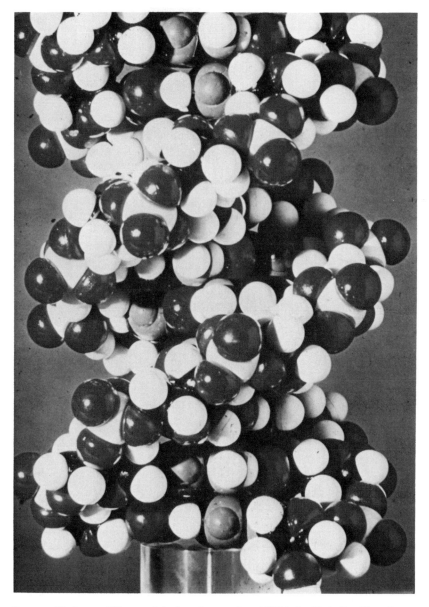

FIGURE 38. Space-filling model of ten base pairs of DNA double helix. The planar base pairs in the center are viewed edge-on, entwined in the two deoxyribose-phosphate "backbones" of the two strands.

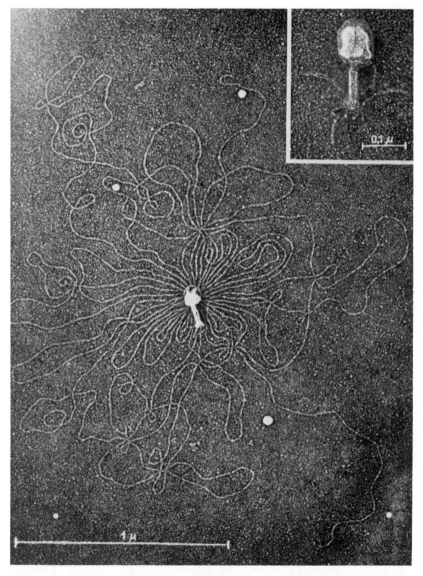

FIGURE 39. The thread-like nature of DNA is better appreciated in this photo-graph of a T-even bacteriophage surrounded by its DNA after osmotic shock. The phage ghost is at center, and the ends of the continuous double-stranded thread of DNA are at top center and bottom right. A human diploid cell contains about 40,000-fold more DNA than this phage or about 2 meters of DNA thread distributed among the 46 chromosomes.

From Kleinschmidt AK, Lang D, Jacherts, D, Zahn, RK: Preparation and length measurements of the total DNA content of T2 bacteriophages. (In German). Biochim Biophys Acta 61:857–864, 1962.

When DNA in solution is heated, the two strands unwind and separate. On subsequent slow cooling the complementary bases reform hydrogen bonds, the strands reassociate, and much of the original double helix reforms. Measurements of the rates of this annealing process give information about the similarity or repetitive nature of base sequences in the DNA. Such measurements indicate that about 60% of the DNA in animal cells is composed of unique sequences. Genes behaving in Mendelian fashion are in this DNA. Another 30% of the total consists of moderately repetitive sequences (ten to several thousand gene copies) coding for histones and for ribosomal RNA, both described in what follows. The highly repetitive DNA making up the remaining 10% consists of short sequences in several thousands of copies that are not transcribed but are found in condensed regions such as the chromomeres of the chromosomes.

CHROMATIN

The chromosomes are composed of chromatin, which is about 15% DNA and 83% protein, histone, and nonhistone. The chromatin (Figure 40) appears to have a structure like a string of beads, with each bead or nucleosome composed of a DNA double helix in a length of 140 base pairs and two molecules of each of four histones. The histones are highly conserved throughout evolution; for example, pea and calf histone H4 are identical except for two conservative amino acid replacements, isoleucine for valine and arginine for lysine.

The DNA in each nucleosome has to be supercoiled or folded to about one seventh its normal length in order to satisfy nucleosome dimensions. The actual DNA structure in nucleosomes is not yet known, but two major models have been advanced on the basis of stereochemical and energetic considerations. One model invokes "kinking" the DNA double helix at regular intervals. The other model smoothly bends the DNA into a superhelix.

Chromatin active in transcription for protein synthesis is called euchromatin. Current evidence indicates that euchromatin exists in the nucleosome structures. Heterochromatin is a condensed form containing DNA not transcribed in the given cell. Structural differences between euchromatin and heterochromatin remain to be completely de-

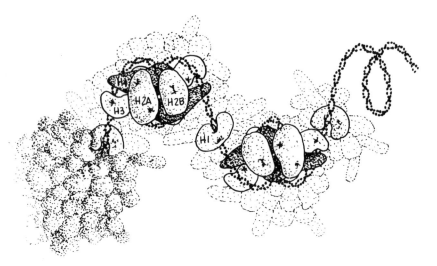

FIGURE 40. In this schematic conception of chromatin, the proteins associated with the DNA at the left are removed in the course from left to right, leaving a bare supercoil of DNA at the right. Each nucleosome consists of 140 base pairs of DNA supercoiled around two molecules each of histones H2A, H2B, H3, and H4. One molecule of histone H1 occupies each spacer region of DNA between the nucleosomes. Spacer DNA has 15 to 100 base pairs, depending on the tissue and species. In addition to these stoichiometric histones, chromatin contains more than 500 other proteins, including contractile and cytoskeletal proteins, nuclear membrane and nuclear pore proteins, nuclear enzymes such as the DNA replicase complex, RNA polymerases, RNA-processing enzymes and RNA binding and transport proteins. The length of DNA in the four nucleosomes and three spacer regions shown here, about 750 base pairs, is sufficient to be the gene for a small protein, of molecular weight about 28,000.

lineated. The nonhistone proteins may play the key role in activity of euchromatin versus heterochromatin.

GENE EXPRESSION

In the process of gene expression (Figure 41), one of the two strands of DNA is transcribed into an RNA of complementary sequence, again according to the rules of base pairing. The RNA whose genetic information is destined to be translated into protein is called mRNA (messenger) and contains a linear sequence of information in the form of units of three purine or pyrimidine residues, each unit specifying an

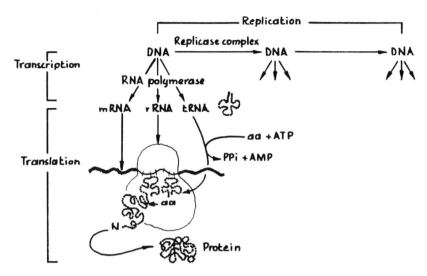

FIGURE 41. An overview of the involvement of DNA in replication and in protein synthesis, involving transcription, then translation. The precise duplication of DNA for cell division is called replication, represented here by the right-pointing arrows. The synthesis of mRNA from the DNA template is called transcription. Protein synthesis involves the translation of the genetic message encoded in the mRNA, a process occurring on the ribosomes and requiring the participation of tRNAs bearing activated amino acids.

amino acid ultimately to be placed in the protein. These three-based units are the codons of the genetic code. The process by which they are translated into a linear sequence of amino acid residues in a protein requires the participation of about 150 different proteins and nucleic acids, including the other two major kinds of RNA, rRNA (ribosomal) and tRNA (transfer). Thus the linear language of DNA is ultimately laid down in a linear sequence of amino acid residues in the protein.

It is this unique sequence in protein that determines three-dimensional structure, and the three-dimensional structure of the protein provides the unique characteristics determining function, whether structural or catalytic. A point mutation changes a single base in a codon. Thus the codon GAG for glutamate in the sixth position of the beta chain of hemoglobin can be changed to GUG, specifying valine. That point mutation produces the valine-for-glutamate substitution known to be the molecular basis for sickle cell disease.

GLOBIN GENES

Because hemoglobin synthesis and structure are so well studied relative to other proteins and because hemoglobin is relevant and familiar in medicine, we might usefully describe gene expression in terms of hemoglobin synthesis insofar as that is possible.

The genes for α globin reside on chromosome 16. Annealing studies reveal two loci or four genes in each diploid cell for α globin. The various forms of α thalassemia are best explained by mutations affecting different numbers of these four genes. Thus in hydrops fetalis all four genes are affected and no α chain exists; in hemoglobin H disease only one of the three genes functions; in thalassemia trait two of four genes work; and in the silent carrier state three of four α globin genes work. These four forms provide another example of gene dose effect.

The genes for γ, δ, and β globins reside on chromosome 11 and are tightly linked, as evident from fusion globins such as $\delta\beta$ in hemoglobin Lepore. Genes δ and β are present at single loci; however, two loci for γ genes exist in tandem, producing γ globins differing only at position 136, one having a glycine residue and one having an alanine residue.

DIRECTION IN DNA, RNA, AND PROTEIN

Single strands of DNA and RNA have a direction, just as these words before you. The ends of the strands are designated 5' and 3' after the pentose carbon atoms not involved in phosphodiester bonds. Thus in shorthand a single strand of DNA or RNA can be depicted

$$AGC$$
$$5' \quad \text{\\\\} \quad 3'$$

in which the letters designate the base residues, adenine, guanine, and cytosine; the vertical lines symbolize ribose or deoxyribose residues; and the diagonal lines stand for phosphate residues. Of the three phosphate residues shown, the 5' one is a monoester, whereas the others are diesterified. An even briefer shorthand for this trinucleotide is pApGpC. Removal of the 5′ phosphate residue gives ApGpC, and attachment of a 3′ phosphate residue gives ApGpCp. In all cases the direction of the trinucleotide is the same. A shorter notation omits the p's, thus AGC.

New DNA is synthesized in the 5′ to 3′ direction by DNA polymerase according to base-pairing instructions in the existing complementary or template strand, which has the opposite orientation, thus is antiparallel:

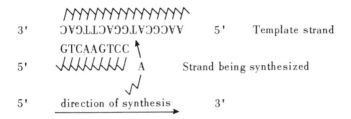

3′	ɔⱯƆꞱꞱƆⱯƆƆꞱⱯƆƆƆⱯⱯ	5′	Template strand
5′	GTCAAGCC		
			Strand being synthesized
5′	direction of synthesis	3′	

Similarly, RNA polymerases synthesize RNA in the 5′ to 3′ direction according to the base sequence in the antiparallel template strand of DNA. That strand is the "sense" strand of DNA, because it alone is a template for RNA synthesis at that location. The direction of DNA and RNA is directly related to the direction of proteins. Thus the 5′ end of a mRNA corresponds to the amino end of a protein, and the 3′ end of a mRNA corresponds to the carboxy terminal of a protein. By convention, 5′ and amino ends are written to the left, and 3′ and carboxy groups are written to the right. Thus in the codon, AUG, the adenylate residue is 5′ and the guanylate residue is 3′. The message AUGUCACAG specifies the tripeptide Met–Ser–Arg, in which methionine is at the amino and arginine at the carboxy terminal.

TRANSCRIPTION

Globin genes are transcribed by an enzyme called RNA polymerase II. The enzyme uses ribonucleoside triphosphates (ATP, GTP, UTP, and CTP) as substrates to synthesize a single strand of mRNA complementary to the sense strand of the DNA in the globin gene being transcribed. Other RNA polymerases are used to synthesize the types of RNA that are not subsequently translated into protein. Thus RNA polymerase I is localized in the nucleolus and is responsible for synthesis of 18S and 28S rRNA. RNA polymerase III is located in the nucleoplasm with RNA polymerase II and synthesizes tRNA and the 5S rRNA.

When RNA polymerase II transcribes a globin gene, the initial product is a precursor of globin mRNA. The precursor is in a class called heterogeneous nuclear RNA (HnRNA). The precursor is modified in at least two ways before passage into the cytoplasm: At the 5' end of the precursor a "cap" is added, and at the 3' end a stretch of 50 to 75 adenylate residues is added. The "cap" consists of a GTP residue in 5'–5' linkage and of methylation of the 5' terminal bases. The precise function of the cap and poly A segments remains to be learned.

Modification of precursor for globin mRNA may be even more extensive. Recent evidence reveals that the gene for β globin and probably many or most mammalian genes contain spacers that do not ultimately appear in mRNA. A spacer of 450 base pairs is found in the middle of the mouse β globin gene. Thus the spacer or insert is as large as the gene itself. Yet unclear is whether (1) the spacer is transcribed into precursor of mRNA, then removed; (2) the spacer is skipped over by RNA polymerase, thus never appearing in mRNA; or (3) the mRNA is synthesized in two pieces lacking the spacer sequence with subsequent joining of the pieces.

In the cases of globin and of ovalbumin, another protein whose gene has spacers, the purpose and function of the spacers are not evident. However, in the case of immunoglobulins, a role for gene spacers is more easily imagined. Available evidence indicates that the constant and the variable regions of immunoglobulin heavy and light chains have separate genes. Thus in the case of light chains, two genes would designate a single polypeptide chain. Early supporting evidence came from immunoglobulin sequence studies. In a patient with monoclonal overproduction of light chains, as in multiple myeloma, and with the rare concomitant overproduction of heavy chains by another malignant clone, the constant regions of the light and heavy chains were different, as expected, but the variable regions had an identical sequence. The same situation pertained in several other patients reported subsequently. The simplest explanation for this finding is that the same variable-region gene was used by both malignant clones in construction of the overproduced monoclonal heavy and light chains, and that different constant-region genes were used. Now direct sequencing of mouse immunoglobulin genes has confirmed and extended the concept of multiple genes for a single polypeptide chain. The DNA for a single light chain of mouse immunoglobulin begins with a leader sequence, which codes for a segment of polypeptide believed to be necessary for transport of the finished protein and destined to be removed. Following the leader sequence in the DNA is a 93-base spacer, then a sequence coding for amino acid residues 1 through 98, the V region in the light chain. Residues 99 through 112 are encoded in a stretch of DNA called the J (Joining) region, from a part of the genome distant from the V region in embryonic DNA but juxtaposed in mature cells producing immunoglobulins. Following the J region is a spacer of about 1,250 bases, then the DNA sequence for the C region of the immunoglobulin light chain. The J region may generate antibody diversity by mediating variable joining of the DNA sequences for V and C regions of the light chains. Other mechanisms are necessary to explain the 1,000 different light chains and 1,000 different heavy chains needed to provide 1,000,000 different IgG molecules, considered a minimum estimate of antibody diversity. Leading hypotheses include the existence of large numbers of variable region genes, and the increase in diversity of these genes by somatic mutation and by crossover events mediated by similar bases in and near spacer DNA.

Even without the spacer, globin RNA is much larger than the 438 base residues required to encode 146 amino acid residues. Both the 5' and the 3' ends have untranslated regions of unknown function. The 3' untranslated region is highly conserved in various species. This region is 132 bases in length and becomes of clinical interest in hemoglobins Icaria and Constant Spring, both having α globins 172 residues long, because of a mutation in the termination codon. In these hemoglobins the extra amino acids are placed according to information in the 3' sequence not ordinarily translated.

In summary globin mRNA can be depicted

5'–Cap–Untranslated— AUG–Translated–Spacer(s)–Translated–UAA
–Untranslated–Poly A–3'

AUG is the initiator codon, and UAA is the terminator codon for translation, the process by which the transcribed genetic message is "read out" into protein. An orthochromatic erythroblast contains about 20,000 globin mRNA molecules.

A typical mammalian cell contains about 12,000 different mRNA molecules. About 10,000 of these mRNA types are present in only

10–20 copies each. Another 500 mRNAs are more abundant, with several hundred copies, and some 10 or so mRNAs may be present to an extent of 10,000 copies per cell. All groups are shared by various tissues, such as liver, kidney, and brain, but in differing relative abundances. Thus albumin mRNA present in 10,000 copies in a liver cell might have only 10 copies in a kidney cell. Kidney cells are known to synthesize albumin at very low levels. The known levels of several specific liver enzymes are calculated to be maintainable by as few as 1–10 mRNA molecules per cell.

Implicit in the foregoing discussion of DNA replication and of transcription is the ability of certain proteins to recognize certain sequences of DNA, for example starting points. The structure of DNA leaves little to recognize other than specific base-pair sequences. Interesting types of these sequences called palindromes are located at many critical recognition points in DNA. In language, a palindrome is a letter sequence reading the same in either direction, for example,

Able was I ere I saw Elba or *A man, a plan, a canal, Panama.*

In DNA a palindrome is a base pair sequence with a twofold radial axis of symmetry. For example the base-pair sequence

would read the same way if rotated 180° around an axis perpendicular to this page, shown as a dot. A property of palindromes which may explain their presence at recognition sites in DNA is their ability to loop out by base pairing with part of the sequence on the same strand rather than on the complementary strand. Thus,

The cleavage sites recognized by restriction endonucleases are palindromes. These endonucleases are discussed under "DNA replacement" in the final chapter.

The human haploid genome contains an estimated 2,000,000 palindromes of average length 190 nucleotidyl residues, widely distributed over all the chromosomes. They comprise about 6% of the human genome. Long palindromes such as these are absent in prokaryotic DNA, and their functions are not fully understood.

TRANSLATION

Translation of the genetic message in mRNA requires the participation of tRNA, ribosomes, and a vast array of associated enzymes. The 70S prokaryotic ribosomes are composed of 30S and 50S subunits, where S is a Svedberg, the unit for sedimentation coefficient. The 30S subunit contains 16S rRNA and 21 proteins, one of which is the binding site for the antibiotic, streptomycin. The wild type E. coli is streptomycin-sensitive, and mutants with single amino-acid changes in this protein are resistant to streptomycin. The 50S subunit contains 5S and 23S rRNA and 34 proteins, one of which is also in the 30S subunit. Another protein in the 50S subunit is peptidyl transferase, the enzyme that catalyzes peptide bond formation in protein synthesis. Eukaryotic ribosomes are larger, 80S, with 40S and 60S subunits containing 18S and 28S rRNA and associated proteins.

The ribosomes recognize a site on the 5' untranslated section of mRNA near the initiator codon, AUG. This ribosome binding site consists of about 10 bases that pair with a complementary sequence at the 3' end of the rRNA in the small subunit. After attachment to the mRNA, each ribosome moves in a 5' to 3' direction along the mRNA in increments of one codon. The process may be usefully divided into the stages initiation, elongation, and termination of protein synthesis.

The initiator codon is ordinarily AUG, specifying methionine. The methionyl residue is carried to the ribosomal site in an activated state, attached to one end of its specific tRNA. The tRNAs are a family of molecules about 80 nucleotidyl residues in length with standard base pairs and unusual hydrogen bonds combining with the base-stacking interactions (seen also in DNA) to give an L-shaped structure. Each tRNA is specific for one and only one of the 20 coded amino acids.

That amino acid is attached to one end of the L after activation by ATP in the reaction

$$\text{Amino acid} + \text{ATP} + \text{tRNA} \rightleftharpoons \text{Aminoacyl–tRNA} + \text{AMP} + \text{PPi}$$

catalyzed by a specific aminoacyl-tRNA synthetase. Thus there is one synthetase for each coded amino acid. At the other end of the L is a sequence of 3 bases complementary and antiparallel to the codon. These bases comprise the anticodon. The interaction of codon and anticodon for methionine may then be written

$$
\begin{array}{c}
{}_3'\diagdown \ \text{CAU} \diagup {}^5, \\
\scriptstyle |\ |\ | \\
5'\diagup \ \text{AUG} \diagdown 3'
\end{array}
$$

This interaction, stabilized on the ribosomal surface, places the initiator or NH_2-terminal amino acid residue in position to interact with the amino acid specified by the next codon. Although there are no "punctuation marks" between the codons, AUG sets the reading frame so that bases are grouped in the correct codons for the entire mRNA. Single base additions or deletions are mutations that change the reading frame.

In elongation, the ribosome then moves from codon to codon in sequence, the essential steps being movement, codon–anticodon matching, and peptide bond formation. As the first ribosome moves away from the early codons, new ribosomes bind at their recognition site, and a single mRNA is read simultaneously by multiple ribosomes, the active complex being a polyribosome. Energy required for the process is supplied by GTP in addition to the ATP used for amino acid activation. Several protein initiation factors and elongation factors are involved, including translocase, an enzyme catalyzing the movement of the ribosome relative to the mRNA. Diphtheria toxin and a toxin of *Pseudomonas aeruginosa* kill by inactivating mammalian translocase. Many antibiotics, including the aminoglycosides, the tetracyclines, and chloramphenicol, exert their antibacterial effects by interfering with various steps in translation.

Termination is triggered by one or more of three codons, UAG, UAA, or UGA, which specify no amino acid and have no complementary tRNA. They are read by release factors, proteins enabling

TABLE 2

The genetic code is universal among species. Each of the 20 coded amino acids, designated by the standard three-letter abbreviation, is genetically specified by a codon. Thus UCA specifies serine, and CUA specifies leucine. Three codons specify termination signals, shown here as "Stop." Some amino acids have six codons (leucine, serine, arginine), whereas tryptophan has only one codon. The codons physically reside in mRNA. The DNA then contains complementary base sequences in its sense strand.

5' BASE	MIDDLE BASE				3' BASE
	U	C	A	G	
	Phe	Ser	Tyr	Cys	U
U	Phe	Ser	Tyr	Cys	C
	Leu	Ser	Stop	Stop	A
	Leu	Ser	Stop	Trp	G
	Leu	Pro	His	Arg	U
C	Leu	Pro	His	Arg	C
	Leu	Pro	Glu	Arg	A
	Leu	Pro	Glu	Arg	G
	Ile	Thr	Asn	Ser	U
A	Ile	Thr	Asn	Ser	C
	Ile	Thr	Lys	Arg	A
	Met	Thr	Lys	Arg	G
	Val	Ala	Asp	Gly	U
G	Val	Ala	Asp	Gly	C
	Val	Ala	Glu	Gly	A
	Val	Ala	Glu	Gly	G

H_2O to hydrolyze the final peptidyl-tRNA bond, releasing the new protein chain. As mentioned earlier, mutation of a terminator codon to a "sense" codon — one specifying an amino acid — results in continuation of translation. In the case of the α globin mRNA, such mutations produce 172-amino acid α globins, their lengths being determined by the position of the next terminator codon in the normally untranslated region before the 5' polyA sequence in globin mRNA.

ASSEMBLY OF SUBUNITS

Hemoglobin has four subunits arranged in a structure of the type $\alpha_2\beta_2$, and each subunit carries the prosthetic group, heme. Thus synthesis of the final product requires an assembly process after folding of each globin subunit. The process is rapid but otherwise not fully understood. Erythroid cells contain small pools of monomers and dimers with heme probably already in place and in equilibrium with the final hemoglobin tetramer. Of course the synthesis of heme must be coordinated with the synthesis of globin, and heme has various controlling effects on the process of globin synthesis. Failure of assembly caused by structural mutations results in degradation of the globin.

PROTEINS MODIFIED AFTER SYNTHESIS

Many proteins are modified after translation (after synthesis of the primary sequence of amino acids). Thus collagen becomes cross-linked, antibodies and other proteins have carbohydrate side chains added, and proinsulin is cleaved to form insulin. Therefore, the final product may be defective not because of a mutation in its own structural gene but because of a mutation in the gene for a modifying enzyme. In such a mechanism we can see one way that different mutations might produce the same clinical disorder, a phenomenon called genetic heterogeneity.

Certain posttranslational modifications produce new amino acids or derivatives. Although only 20 amino acids have codons, as many as 140 derivatives exist in proteins of various species. Thus hydroxyproline and hydroxylysine are amino acid residues in collagen. Recently γ-carboxyglutamic acid residues have been found in human prothrombin and in clotting factors VII, IX, and X. A vitamin-K-dependent liver enzyme places a second carboxyl group on each of ten glutamic acid residues in prothrombin. The resultant γ-carboxyglutamate residues are calcium-ion binding sites essential to clotting. Coumarin anticoagulants block the carboxylation as vitamin K antagonists.

HOW MUTATIONS PRODUCE DISEASE

Through an understanding of the biochemistry of the genetic process we can see some of the ways mutant genes produce disease. A mutation might lead to production of an abnormal RNA or an abnormal protein. Proteins have various functions: For example, collagen is structural, whereas hemoglobin is involved in transport. Others are specific catalysts — the enzymes — and still others are involved in control of genes. The disease resulting from a specific, mutant protein would then illuminate the function of the protein. If localized to a specific amino acid residue in the protein, the mutation might even illuminate the role of that amino acid within the protein. One should expect that mutations in the genes for tRNA and rRNA would have pleiotropic effects, that is, change many phenotypes, because tRNA and rRNA are necessary for the synthesis of all proteins in the cell. The same pleiotropic effects can be expected from mutations in the genes for any of the macromolecules required for protein synthesis and for DNA and RNA synthesis.

HEMOGLOBINOPATHIES

Study of human hemoglobinopathies has enormously illuminated the mechanisms by which point mutations in genes for specific proteins produce disease. Because protein function results from a three-dimensional structure, which in turn is fixed by the sequence of amino acid residues, it then follows that changes in amino acid sequence resulting from mutations would alter protein function. Sickle hemoglobin is one example, and there are more than 100 others for hemoglobin alone. Depending on the position and nature of the amino acid change, the mutant hemoglobin might suffer alteration in solubility (sickle hemoglobin), ability to bind oxygen, stability, or allosteric properties.

Allostery refers to the property of certain proteins consisting of two or more subunits to respond by change in conformation to the binding of specific molecules at distant sites. The changes in conformation have important effects on function. By allostery, a protein becomes able to modify its structure and function in response to signals in the environment. Thus hemoglobin changes its oxygen-binding properties according to pH, CO_2 concentration, 2,3-diphosphoglycerate concentration, and number of oxygen molecules bound. Myoglobin, individual α and β chains, and even β_4 tetramers completely lack these allosteric properties of hemoglobin. Hemoglobins with amino acid replacements at critical contact points between the α and β chains prevent the transmission of conformational changes (allosteric interactions) underlying the cooperativity of oxygen binding, the Bohr effect of protons and CO_2 on oxygen binding, and the effect of diphosphoglycerate on oxygen binding.

Other point mutations in hemoglobin do not primarily affect allosteric interactions. For example, methemoglobinemia, in which the iron in two of the four hemes is permanently in the ferric state, results from a histidine-to-tyrosine change at the positions where histidine normally coordinates with iron. Instead, the negative charge on the ionized tyrosine residue stabilizes the extra positive charge on the iron atom. The ferric heme does not bind oxygen. Such mutations can occur in either the α or β chains.

In hemoglobin Hammersmith substitution of a serine residue for a phenylalanine residue causes the heme to bind less securely to the globin. In hemoglobin Riverdale an arginine-for-glycine change impedes proper folding of the hemoglobin, because the arginine residue is too large to fit, and the hemoglobin is unstable.

THALASSEMIAS

Several of the diseases grouped with the thalassemias (Figure 42) best illustrate the clinical results of mutations of regulatory genes as distinct from mutations within the globin genes themselves. In these thalassemias, the globins are structurally normal, but are produced in diminished amounts. Because of the $\alpha_2\beta_2$ subunit structure of hemoglobin, balanced synthesis of α and β globins is essential. In β thalassemias, β globin is decreased or absent. As a result α globin accumulates and precipitates in erythroid cells, damaging the cell membranes and interfering with erythropoiesis. In α thalassemia, α globin is decreased or absent. The β globin now in relative excess, forms β_4 tetramers

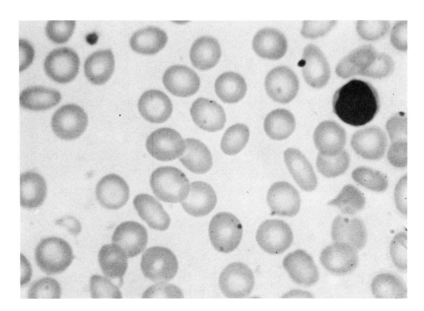

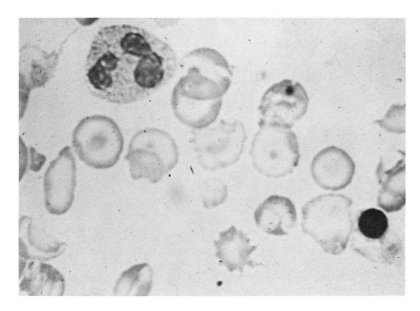

FIGURE 42. Thalassemic red blood cell changes. In the heterozygote (thalassemia minor) some β globin synthesis occurs, and the blood smear (top) shows mild to moderate anisocytosis, poikilocytosis, and hypochromia. The $\beta°$ thalassemic blood smear (bottom) shows severe hypochromia, anisocytosis, and poikilocytosis.

called hemoglobin H, which eventually precipitates to give inclusions leading to hemolysis.

Two genetic features of thalassemia mutations are their tight linkages to the genes for the globins and their cis activity: they affect only the globin structural gene(s) on the same chromosome, not the homologous chromosome of the pair. Thus a patient with the sickle mutation in the β globin gene on one chromosome 11 and with a β thalassemia mutation on the other chromosome 11 would produce normal amounts of β^s globin and decreased amounts of β globin. The tight linkage of thalassemia genes to globin genes is demonstrated by the observation that in progeny of such double heterozygotes for hemoglobinopathies and thalassemia no crossover event has ever been detected.

The reason for decreased α globin in the α thalassemias is simply gene deletion of one or more of the four α-globin genes, as already mentioned. In the β thalassemias, a more complicated situation exists, implicating mutations in controlling sequences near the β globin gene. The simplest case is homozygous persistence of fetal hemoglobin ($\alpha_2\gamma_2$), in which total absence of β globin synthesis results from total deletion of the β globin gene. However, in some cases of β^0 thalassemia, the β globin genes are present, but no β globin mRNA is synthesized. Here the defect is in control of transcription, possibly because of the absence of a promoter site (binding site for RNA polymerase) just before the β globin gene. In other cases of β^0 thalassemia, β globin mRNA is present but is not properly translated. Here the defect might lie in the ribosome binding site in the 5' untranslated region of the β globin mRNA. Thus some clinical situations are ultimately best explained by mutations in regulatory regions of DNA coding for initiation signals controlling transcription or translation.

In the thalassemias, we see another example of genetic heterogeneity: Mutations affecting different levels of protein synthesis, transcription, or translation give the same end result—absence of a gene product.

DIFFERENTIATION

Every normal human cell contains genes for the α and β chains of hemoglobin, but only in certain erythropoietic cells are those genes expressed. Cell differentiation is a consequence of differential gene expression. We know that even in simple bacterial cells, all of the genes are not expressed, and moreover, that the rate of protein synthesis from any given gene varies over a wide range.

Some genes encode proteins whose function is to inhibit or enhance the rate of transcription of other genes. For example, one such repressor protein apparently combines with heme to turn off the gene encoding δ aminolevulinic acid synthetase, the first enzyme in the pathway of heme biosynthesis. In acute intermittent porphyria, the normal level of feedback repression does not occur. The consequent increase in the aminolevulinic acid synthetase leads to the overproduction of aminolevulinic acid and porphobilinogen. Almost nothing is understood about specific gene control in human cells and the extrapolation of such regulatory mechanisms to the elucidation of tissue and organ differentiation. However, elegant studies in bacterial model systems have provided a sound basis for this exciting area.

CONTROL OF GENE EXPRESSION

Two means of control of gene expression in mammalian cells deserve mention. In one the rate of transcription of a gene is affected by glucocorticoids. The mouse mammary tumor virus is an RNA tumor virus that exists as a DNA provirus in the genome of its host, as discussed in the next chapter. Actually multiple copies of the provirus are integrated into the mouse DNA. Treatment of mouse cells, bearing the provirus, with a glucocorticoid specifically increases the rate of mouse mammary tumor virus RNA synthesis, or transcription, about tenfold. The steroid binds to a cytoplasmic protein receptor, and this steroid–receptor complex then enters the nucleus and recognizes specific genes. The mechanisms of recognition and stimulation of transcription are not understood, but already the regulation of genes by steroids has achieved clinical usefulness, as in the treatment of hereditary angioneurotic edema with attenuated androgens (final chapter).

The second example is gene multiplication or gene amplification as a means of increasing the output of a gene product. Some of the mouse cells treated with methotrexate become highly resistant to the drug. One basis for this resistance is a selective multiplication of the gene for dihydrofolate reductase, the enzyme inhibited by the drug. The gene amplification is accompanied by proportional increases in mRNA for dihydrofolate reductase and in the enzyme itself. The gene multiplication can reach levels of 200-fold. This mechanism may be at play in human cancer cells that become resistant to methotrexate, for such cells regularly contain increased levels of dihydrofolate reductase. In this phenomenon and others to be discussed in the next chapter, we see that the mammalian genome may be subjected to important changes in content.

In such gene amplification are the extra gene copies chromosomal or nonchromosomal? Unequal sister chromatid exchange would provide a mechanism for tandem gene duplications in a chromosome. However, the extrachromosomal amplification of ribosomal genes in amphibian oocytes is a precedent for the other mechanism in differentiation and development.

GENETICS AND CANCER

MUTATIONS CAUSE CANCER

The relationship of cancer to genetics is observable at the chromosomal and Mendelian levels and is now becoming understood in molecular terms. All levels of observation point to the concept that most
cancers result from somatic cell mutations. The important possible
exception, experimental mouse teratocarcinoma, is mentioned at the
end of this chapter.

Certain cancers or diseases predisposing to cancer occur with simple
Mendelian pedigrees. Thus, retinoblastoma, neurofibromatosis, and
familial adenomatous colonic polyposis (Figure 43) are autosomal dominant in mode of inheritance, and xeroderma pigmentosum and certain
Wilms' tumors are autosomal recessive. Other cancers may show increased incidence in certain families but not show clearly Mendelian
pedigrees, and these cancers might best be explained by the action of
environmental factors on a polygenic system.

CHROMOSOMAL MARKERS

Some cancers have chromosomal markers. For example, the Philadelphia chromosome (Ph^1) in chronic myelogenous leukemia is the
remnant of a major translocation from the long arm of one chromosome
22. The material lost by chromosome 22 is translocated to the distal
end of the long arm of another autosome, usually number 9. Presence
of the Philadelphia chromosome has been observed before onset of the
disease. The translocation appears to be acquired, for it was found in
a leukemic patient whose monozygotic twin had neither the disease
nor the Philadelphia chromosome. Meningiomas frequently lack one

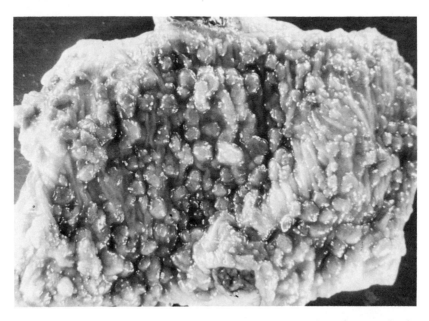

FIGURE 43. In familial adenomatous colonic polyposis, benign adenomas begin to appear at an average age of 24 years. The lesions are confined to the colon and rectum and average 1000 in number. Even in the short segment shown here the adenomas are too numerous to count easily. Rectal bleeding and diarrhea begin in the middle 30's ordinarily, but the age range is enormous, from early childhood to old age. Adenocarcinoma appears virtually without exception and often at multiple sites. Prophylactic colectomy is indicated. Often the rectum can be spared with adequate surveillance and early treatment for any cancer developing. Because of the autosomal dominant mode of inheritance, children of affected people must be followed closely.

chromosome 22. Some cases of retinoblastoma have a characteristic deletion of the long arm of one chromosome 13 (13q–). African Burkitt lymphoma usually has an extra band in the long arm of chromosome 14. In other cancers, such as the acute leukemias, chromosomal abnormalities are usually present but are not specific.

Chromosomes can be used as markers in male-female homografts: a girl with acute lymphoblastic leukemia was given 1,000 rads wholebody irradiation followed by an infusion of marrow from her HLA-matched brother. The leukemia recurred 62 days after the graft in the XY cells, a result supporting the concept of a leukemogenic agent present in the girl and capable of infecting fresh cells from her brother.

TUMOR ORIGIN

Characterization of G6PD in heterozygous females with tumors has been used to determine whether various human tumors arise from a single cell (clonal origin) or from multiple cells. Several females with chronic myelogenous leukemia (CML) had both types A and B G6PD in cultured fibroblasts and were, therefore, heterozygotes. However, all of their leukemic granulocytes were of either type A or B G6PD but not both. Therefore, their leukemias arose from single cell precursors rather than from many cells or from cell-to-cell spread, as by a virus. Other malignant tumors give the same result, including Burkitt's lymphoma, of particular interest because of its viral etiology. The test revealed that polycythemia vera has a clonal stem cell origin for its increased numbers of circulating erythrocytes, granulocytes, and platelets. Therefore, the disease is neoplastic.

Interesting tumors of multiclonal origin are the neurofibromas in hereditary neurofibromatosis and breast carcinoma, which may be hormone-dependent. In these cases, we can easily imagine mechanisms for multiclonal origin.

DISEASES OF FAULTY GENETIC REPAIR

Four diseases inherited in the autosomal recessive mode are characterized by inability to repair diverse genetic damage and by early development of malignancies: xeroderma pigmentosum, Bloom's syndrome, Fanconi's pancytopenia, and ataxia telangiectasia (Louis-Barr syndrome). In xeroderma pigmentosum (Figure 44) the defect lies in an enzyme responsible for excision of mutations, such as thymine dimers caused by ultraviolet light, from the damaged DNA (Figure 45). Consequently, the disease is characterized by sun-induced acceleration of the aging of skin with ultimate skin cancer of all types.

The other three diseases all exhibit chromosomal abnormalities such as gaps, breaks, and rearrangements. In ataxia telangiectasia, the lymphocytes develop translocations involving the long arm of chromosome 14, a finding of particular interest because of the relation of chromosome 14 to Burkitt's lymphoma. The most characteristic ab-

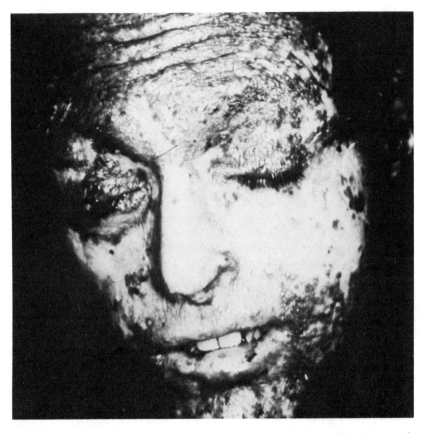

FIGURE 44. In end-stage xeroderma pigmentosum sun-exposed skin bears multiple cancers, the final result of inability to repair somatic mutations caused by sunlight.

erration in Bloom's syndrome is a quadriradial, representing the partial pairing of chromatids of homologous chromosomes. Such configurations are involved in the crossing over or exchange of chromatids between homologous chromosomes, a process undoubtedly occurring by the same mechanism as sister chromatid exchange (Figure 46). Sister chromatid exchange is increased tenfold in Bloom's syndrome, and the frequency of homologous chromatid exchange in quadriradials must also be increased. Tissues with high mitotic indices are particularly susceptible to cancer in Bloom's syndrome. How could increased

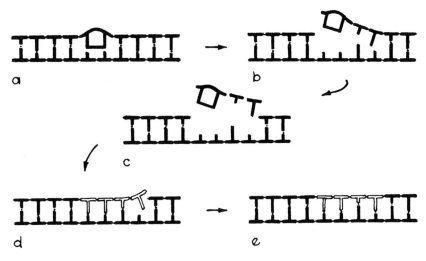

FIGURE 45. Repair of DNA damaged by ultraviolet light. (a) Two adjacent thymine residues on one strand of a DNA double helix have been covalently linked
by action of ultraviolet light. The thymine dimer distorts the normal geometry
of the double helix and interferes with proper base pairing. This is the physical
basis for one type of mutation. (b) An endonuclease has recognized the mutation
and has started repair by cleaving the phosphodiester backbone. In xeroderma
pigmentosum this endonuclease is missing or defective. (c) An exonuclease continues the removal of the thymine dimer and surrounding nucleotidyl residues.
(d) A DNA polymerase replaces the excised residues according to base-pairing
rules and information in the template strand of the DNA. Finally, ligase forms
the final phosphodiester bond to complete the repair.

homologous chromatid exchange lead to cancer? An interesting hypothesis has been proposed: After homologous chromatid exchange,
two of the four possible segregation patterns for the recombinant chromosomes would yield chromosomes homozygous at loci that were heterozygous before the change. If genes at these loci are related to the
development of cancer, their homozygous presence could trigger malignancy in those particular daughter cells.

Normally, sister chromatid exchange signals the operation of a DNA
repair mechanism. When normal cells are exposed to alkylating agents
that cross-link DNA, the number of sister chromatid exchanges increases dramatically. Lymphocytes from patients with Fanconi's anemia do not give this response, a finding that suggests a defect in some
DNA repair mechanism in this disease.

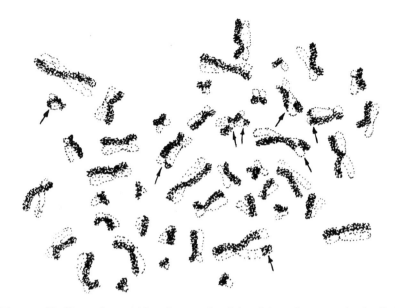

FIGURE 46. Sister chromatid exchange. Special staining after growth of cells in medium containing bromodeoxyuridine in place of thymine differentiates the old from the new chromatids on each chromosome. Therefore, points of crossover between sister chromatids are clearly seen.

Although these four diseases of defective genetic repair are rare, their importance in relation to cancer is more than academic: according to the Hardy–Weinberg law, heterozygotes for ataxia–telangiectasia comprise about 1% of the American population and may account for more than 5% of cancer deaths before age 45.

VIRUSES AND CANCER

Cells cultured from patients with Fanconi's pancytopenia have, in addition to chromosomal abnormalities, a greatly increased susceptibility to transformation by SV40 virus. Currently enormous research attention has been focused on the possible viral etiology of human cancer.

Cell transformation by a virus is a test used to determine the potential of the virus to cause cancer. The virus is placed on cells being maintained in tissue culture. Transformed cells have a permanent, genetic change causing them to grow uncontrollably in tissue culture: that is, to pile up and grow not as a monolayer but as a densely packed colony. A second characteristic of transformed cells is their ability to become malignant tumors when injected into the animal of origin. No virus isolated from a human tumor has yet been found to cause transformation of human cells in tissue culture.

In animals, the viruses causing cancer can be RNA viruses or DNA viruses. In man, the viruses more closely associated with cancer are the DNA viruses. The adenoviruses comprise one type of DNA virus. There are 31 adenoviruses known to infect man, and of those 31, 13 either transform animal cells or cause cancer in animals or both. Thus 13 of 31 adenoviruses that infect man cause cancer in other animals, but none of these adenoviruses has been found to transform human cells in tissue culture.

Recent experiments have shown that only one viral gene is required to transform a cell. Small segments of adenovirus DNA, equivalent to single genes, have been detected in human tumors, but such detection does not implicate the virus in the causation of the tumor.

Adenovirus 12, which is strongly oncogenic in hamsters, is a respiratory pathogen in man and is found in human feces. However, tests that would detect 2% the adenovirus DNA per tumor cell revealed none in more than 150 human tumors examined. In contrast, hamster tumors contain multiple copies of the causative adenovirus 12 genome.

EPSTEIN-BARR VIRUS

Herpes viruses are closest of all to the problem of cancer in man. Epstein-Barr virus or EB virus is a herpes virus that causes Burkitt's lymphoma (Figure 47) and infectious mononucleosis and that may cause nasopharyngeal carcinoma. The virus is present both in a free form and integrated into the genome of Burkitt's lymphoma cells and is carried in poorly differentiated nasopharyngeal carcinoma cells. The virus infects the majority of adults in all countries. From those people who are seropositive for Epstein-Barr virus, lymphoid cell lines carrying Epstein-Barr virus DNA and Epstein-Barr virus nuclear antigen can be established in culture. A fascinating and undoubtedly significant

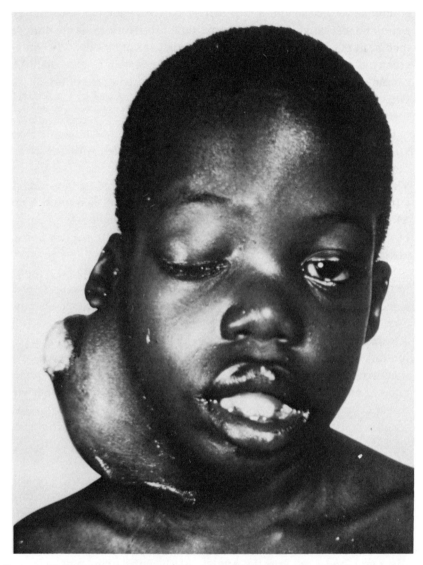

FIGURE 47. Burkitt's lymphoma is a lymphosarcoma accounting for half of all childhood tumors in parts of Africa with high rainfall and temperature, near the equator. The disease also occurs in children of other races and in other countries. It typically arises in the maxilla or mandible and frequently involves other organs, especially ovaries and kidneys with relative sparing of lymph nodes and spleen. Spontaneous regression may occur, and response to chemotherapy is good with frequent apparent cure as in this case after this photograph was made.

difference between these nonmalignant cells carrying the Epstein-Barr virus and the Burkitt's lymphoma cells is that the latter contain a specific extra band at the distal end of one chromosome 14 in almost every case. Americans with lymphoma do not have Epstein-Barr virus DNA or nuclear antigen in those lymphomas. Thus, the Epstein-Barr virus is specific for Burkitt's lymphoma.

In what is probably a new immunodeficiency disease, males inherit in an X-linked recessive mode the inability to cope normally with EB virus infection. These males either succumb from infectious mononucleosis or from agammaglobulinemia or from B-cell lymphoma. What locus on the X chromosome controls this response, how it works, and what relation it bears to other X-linked immune deficient disorders are unanswered questions. However, we see here the intricate interaction of genetic and environmental factors in the production of cancer. In addition, we see an environmental factor, EB virus, becoming a genetic factor through actual incorporation into the genome of somatic cells.

According to a recent hypothesis, resistance to tumors caused by Epstein-Barr virus (but not resistance to infectious mononucleosis) has been essential for man's evolution in the presence of this virus. In contrast, resistance to spontaneous tumors, which commonly appear after the reproductive years, is not fixed by selection, being unnecessary to survival of the species. Laboratory tumors produced by highly oncogenic viruses may not even remotely resemble spontaneous "natural" tumors, which evolve in the host to resist all control mechanisms, including the immunological. The bearers of such tumors are probably normal immunologically, not deficient.

The other herpes virus linked with cancer is herpes virus type 2, which causes genital infections thought by many to be linked epidemiologically to carcinoma of the cervix.

RNA TUMOR VIRUSES

RNA tumor viruses are found in a wide variety of vertebrates but have never been isolated from man. The major group is called Type C. Some —for example, Rous sarcoma virus—are among the most potent carcinogens known, whereas others do not produce cancer. RNA tumor viruses contain about sixfold more RNA (genetic information) than poliomyelitis virus. They contain an enzyme, RNA-dependent DNA polymerase or reverse transcriptase, capable of synthesizing an exact DNA copy of their RNA genomes. The discovery of that enzyme revolutionized concepts of the direction of flow for genetic information, previously believed always to be from DNA to RNA to protein. Moreover, RNA tumor viruses contain at least three other enzymes with the combined capability of placing the provirus DNA synthesized by their reverse transcriptases into the host genome. After infection of mammalian cells by such RNA tumor viruses one can show the new virogenes to be in the host genome. By itself the existence of a virogene in the genome of a cell is not sufficient to cause cancer. What other factors are involved are unresolved.

When virogene DNA resides in cells of the germ line, its replication during cell division provides for vertical transmission. When it resides in somatic cells, its being copied in the conventional fashion (DNA to RNA) provides new viruses capable of horizontal transmission to neighboring cells. Feline leukemia virus is horizontally transmitted among cats, and the four fatal diseases it causes make it the greatest killer of pet cats.

The mouse mammary tumor virus exemplifies type B RNA tumor viruses, which are less common than type C. Such viruses are bigger than type C and have an eccentric nucleoid. Baby mice receive this virus in their father's semen, in the mother's ovum, from their mother's milk, and finally within the genomes donated by both the mother and the father. Thus, a newborn mouse receives this virus intact from both the mother and the father and in addition receives a DNA copy of the virus which has been incorporated into the genome of the mother and of the father. A virus with the same morphological characteristics has been found in human milk. This virus from human milk produces a DNA hybridizing with mouse mammary tumor virus but not with mouse type C leukemia virus.

Normal, uninfected cells contain DNA sequences and protein antigens also present in RNA tumor viruses. Temin's protovirus hypothesis holds that a normal cellular system of genetic information transfer from DNA to RNA to DNA, originally a basis for cellular differentiation, evolved to produce RNA particles wrapped in the necessary proteins for horizontal transmission of genetic information. These particles are our present RNA "tumor" viruses, according to the theory, and they exist in a sort of equilibrium between the free virus and that incorporated as DNA into the host's genome.

CARCINOGENS AND MUTAGENS

Currently enormous emphasis is placed on environmental carcinogens. At first glance the emphasis on environment might tend to diminish the importance of genetic factors in cancer. However, we must ask by what mechanism does an environmental carcinogen work? The Ames test for carcinogens now has clearly shown that almost all carcinogens are mutagens. Thus chemicals join radiation and viruses as environmental agents that produce cancer by genetic mechanisms. The Ames test has, parenthetically, produced some specific surprises; for example, nitrofurantoin is a potent mutagen!

Sometimes the genetic element precedes the environmental factor in carcinogenesis. Thus lung cancer has been so strongly linked to cigarette smoking that genetic predisposition was at first overlooked. We now know that people differ in levels of the enzyme, aryl hydrocarbon hydroxylase, inherited according to Mendelian rules. The enzyme hydroxylates aryl hydrocarbons in cigarette smoke, thereby changing them into more potent carcinogens. People able to produce high levels of this enzyme may be more likely to develop lung cancer from a given amount of smoking than people with low levels.

Whatever the specific causative agent, and whatever the level of observation available now, most cancer seems ultimately to result from a change or changes in DNA. However, elegant studies of mouse teratocarcinoma cells have furnished an example of a nonmutational basis for transformation to malignancy and reversal to normalcy. When such cells were injected into mouse embryos at the blastocyst stage and followed by means of genetic markers, the cancer cells developed into a variety of completely normal tissues, even contributing to a germ line forming normal sperm. In this case the cancer cells appear to be totipotential and programmed for cancer on a nonhereditary basis somehow determined by their milieu.

TREATMENT OF GENETIC DISEASE

Too frequently genetic diseases are considered hopeless and attackable only by prevention or by a general supportive treatment. Resistance to the idea that hereditary factors may contribute to the etiology of mental disease has been based partly on the notion that hereditary components cannot be treated. However, treatment is available for many genetic disorders, and research is constantly developing specific treatment. What follows is only a representative sampling.

SURGERY FOR PHENOTYPE

A framework for discussion of treatment can be built into our concepts of genotype and phenotype. From the discussion of biochemical genetics, we now understand an abnormal genotype as a lesion in DNA structure and an abnormal phenotype as the result of abnormal protein function. Alteration of phenotype by surgery can dramatically improve health if not "cure" genetic diseases such as retinoblastoma, cleft lip and palate, club foot, pyloric stenosis, hypospadias, congenital heart defects, and hereditary spherocytosis (Figure 48).

MOLECULAR THERAPY

Abnormal enzyme function is usually manifest by the accumulation of excess substrate or by the lack of product. (Rarely, a defective enzyme is *more* efficient than the normal counterpart and produces too much product, as in the case of a mutant phosphoribosyl pyrophosphate synthetase that produces too much PRPP and causes a rare form of

96

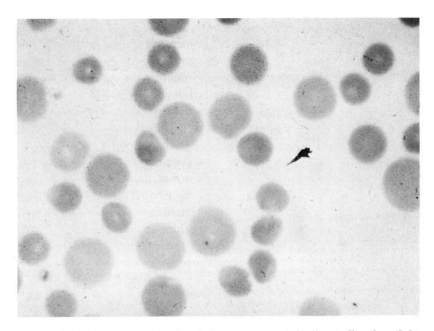

FIGURE 48. Hereditary spherocytosis is an autosomal dominant disorder of the red blood cell membrane with increased permeability and a resultant spheroidal shape, evident in this blood smear. The spleen is the only organ removing spherocytes, producing anemia, jaundice, and splenomegaly. Splenectomy restores red blood cell survival to normal and is in effect curative.

gout.) Therefore, attack on genetic diseases can be directed at removal of excess substrate, provision of missing products, provision of cofactors to bolster activity of ailing enzymes, structural alteration of enzymes, replacement of enzymes, or replacement of DNA. The last three of these approaches are still highly experimental, and replacement of DNA (genetic engineering) has been the focus of great excitement and controversy.

CHANGING METABOLISM WITH DRUGS

To illustrate the approaches listed, I shall mention some rare diseases. Hopefully the approaches will serve as prototypes for more common diseases. But first let us consider a treatment we use to alter the course of a common genetic disease complex, gout (Figure 49). In the various forms of gout characterized by overproduction of uric acid and with intact hypoxanthine–guanine phosphoribosyl transferase (HGPRTase, the purine-salvage enzyme defective in Lesch-Nyhan disease) we treat with the hypoxanthine analog, allopurinol. The allopurinol is converted by HGPRTase to the ribonucleotide, which participates in feedback inhibition of amidotransferase, the first committed enzyme in de novo uric acid synthesis. In addition, allopurinol depletes cells of phosphoribosyl pyrophosphate in becoming the ribonucleotide, thereby decreasing further the activity of amidotransferase, which is substrate-limited. Finally, allopurinol inhibits xanthine oxidase. The use of the drug is a superb example of and model for specific interference with metabolic processes under genetic control.

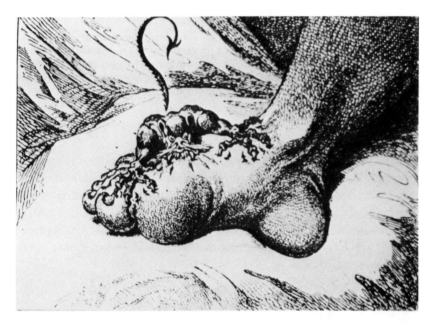

FIGURE 49. The agony of acute gouty arthritis was likened to the "gnawing of a dog" by Thomas Sydenham in his famous Treatise on the Gout (1683). Here James Gillray (1799) is perhaps depicting that description. This genetically heterogeneous disease is treatable by specific alteration of purine metabolism with allopurinol.

The elevated levels of protoporphyrin in blood and skin of patients with protoporphyria produce sensitivity of skin to visible light. Administration of β carotene somehow blocks the sensitization, even though the protoporphyrin levels remain elevated.

REMOVAL OF EXCESS SUBSTRATES

Phenylketonuria and galactosemia are characterized by substrate excess. In phenylketonuria, phenylalanine accumulates because of deficient hydroxylase. The excess phenylalanine interferes with normal development of the central nervous system. By dietary restriction of phenylalanine until maturation of the central nervous system, the disease is successfully treated. In galactosemia galactose, galactose-1-phosphate, and galactitol accumulate because of the absence of galactose-1-phosphate uridyl transferase. The result is mental retardation, cirrhosis, and cataracts. Simple removal of galactose from the diet allows normal growth and development.

PROVIDING MISSING PRODUCTS

As an example of the disease caused by lack of product, orotic aciduria results from a deficiency of two enzymes in the synthetic pathway for uridine-5-phosphate. The failure of growth and development, megaloblastic anemia, and excretion of excessive orotic acid in the urine is cured by the addition of uridine to the diet.

When the missing product is a hormone, simple replacement cures the disease. Thus isolated growth hormone deficiency is treated by administration of human growth hormone, a 188-residue protein which has now been synthesized. Again, L-thyroxine replacement therapy suffices for familial goiter, which results from any one of several defects in the pathway of L-thyroxine synthesis.

VITAMINS FOR COENZYMES

The therapeutic attack can sometimes be directed at the defective enzyme itself rather than at its substrates or products. Some enzymes are defective in coenzyme binding and can be restored to an active state by providing massive concentrations of coenzyme via vitamin therapy. For example, in xanthurenic aciduria, the defective kynureninase does not properly bind its coenzyme, pyridoxal phosphate. When the latter is provided in high levels, the enzyme activity is restored. Therefore, the disease is treated by pharmacologic doses of pyridoxine. The Wernicke-Korsakoff syndrome is a well-known neuropsychiatric disorder that develops from thiamine deficiency in a minority of chronic alcoholics or other malnourished people. This minority has a genetic defect in transketolase. The defective enzyme binds thiamine pyrophosphate, its coenzyme, less avidly than normal. The defect is overcome by therapeutic doses of thiamine. At least 12 other diseases associated with deficiencies of enzymes which require coenzymes can be treated with doses of vitamins ranging from 10 to 100 times the normal requirement. Vitamin-D-resistant rickets is another example.

INDUCTION OF ENZYME SYNTHESIS

Steroid hormones appear to control specific gene expression by transcriptional mechanisms. Thus the attenuated androgen, danazol, is used successfully to induce synthesis of the C1 inhibitor, a protein whose absence causes hereditary angioneurotic edema. Similarly, prednisone effectively treats lysosomal acid phosphatase deficiency by inducing the synthesis of the missing enzyme.

Phenobarbital promptly reverses the chronic jaundice of persons with the Arias type of hyperbilirubinemia. The drug probably works by induction of the glucuronyl transferase, which is low in this autosomal dominant disorder. (The autosomal recessive Crigler-Najjar syndrome is characterized by a defect of the same enzyme and is not reversed by phenobarbital.)

ENZYME MODIFICATION

Another approach involves direct modification of the faulty enzyme or protein. The prototype for permanent, covalent modification of defective proteins to improve function is the carbamylation of sickle hemoglobin with orally administered cyanate. Although the modified hemo-globin has a shifted oxygen-binding curve, and hemoglobin levels rise in treated patients, frequency of sickle crises is not reduced. More-over, the cyanate produces cataracts and peripheral neuropathy in some patients. Nevertheless, the general approach is promising not only for hemoglobinopathies but for enzymatic genetic diseases.

ENZYME REPLACEMENT

Replacement of the defective protein itself is clearly possible when the protein is extracellular, as are the clotting factors. Thus hemophilia A or factor VIII deficiency is now successfully controlled by administra-tion of purified factor VIII. As mentioned earlier, enzyme levels less than 100% may give normal phenotypes. Thus in hemophilia prophy-laxis levels of factor VIII as low as 5% of normal are sufficient to protect against repeated episodes of bleeding.

Replacement of intracellular enzymes is more difficult. However, lysosomal enzymes might be replaceable by exogenous enzymes en-gulfed into pinocytotic vacuoles that merge with lysosomes. Certain genetic diseases, such as Tay-Sachs, Gaucher's and Fabry's diseases and the mucopolysaccharidoses result from deficiencies of lysoso-mal enzymes. For these diseases, direct enzyme replacement remains a possibility to be considered, and Fabry's disease has been treated experimentally with ceramidetrihexosidase purified from human placenta.

In one report, fibroblasts from a galactosemic patient were treated with lambda bacteriophage carrying the gene for galactose-1-phosphate uridyl transferase, and the cells began stable production of the enzyme. However, the cells were in tissue culture where they could be treated with a ratio of bacteriophage to cell in the range of 1,000 to 10,000, clearly not applicable to the whole organism.

Shope papilloma virus elevates the arginase level in infected epithe-lial cells. Workers researching the virus apparently carry a benign, lifelong infection and have low levels of arginine in the blood. Some initial success has been reported in lowering arginine levels in the blood of children with hyperargininemia after infecting them with the virus.

DNA REPLACEMENT

Finally, I should mention what has popularly come to be known as genetic engineering. The term refers to the new ability of scientists to isolate DNA pieces containing selected genes and to insert such DNA into the genomes of other species. For example, with this methodology scientists constructed a new genome consisting of SV40 viral DNA (SV40 produces tumors in apes), about 10% of λ bacteriophage DNA, and the galactose operon of *Escherichia coli*. This work raised the question of whether viruses producing tumors in mammals could be introduced into *E. coli*, then spread widely via the *E. coli* only to subsequently emerge and produce tumors in the mammalian host of the *E. coli*. The dangers of this experimentation were considered sufficient for the Committee on Recombinant DNA Molecules of the National Academy of Sciences to call a voluntary moratorium. The moratorium is now ended and research is continuing under strict NIH guidelines.

The essential methodology (Figure 50) involves the use of restriction endonucleases, bacterial enzymes that recognize and cleave DNA at palindromic sequences. For example, the Eco RI endonuclease cleaves DNA as shown by the arrows at any and every base-pair sequence

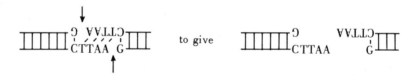

The resulting DNA fragments are double stranded with single stranded –TTAA ends capable of base pairing to complementary "sticky ends" on the other fragments. Any DNA cleaved in this way, regardless of the species of origin, can be annealed to any other DNA fragments resulting from the same kind of cleavage. After annealing of the fragments, an enzyme called DNA ligase reconstitutes the covalent links to give intact phosphodiester chains as in the original DNA. DNA fragments made by restriction endonucleases can thus be incorporated into plasmid DNA and carried by the plasmid DNA into bacteria.

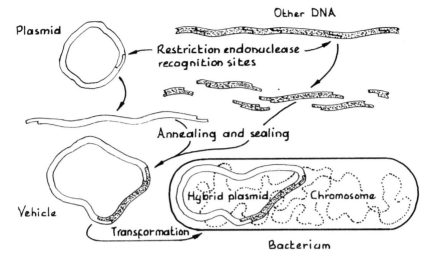

FIGURE 50. DNA from one species can be covalently attached by DNA from any other species with the help of one of an array of restriction endonucleases, now commercially available. Here one DNA is a plasmid able to infect a bacterium and thereby to introduce the foreign DNA into the bacterium.

Plasmids are molecules of DNA that exist in bacterial cells and replicate independently of the bacterial genome. Frequently they carry genes conferring antibiotic resistance, a phenotype that can be used to select bacterial clones bearing plasmids. A hybrid plasmid carries a piece of foreign DNA and can be cloned in a bacterium. Multiple copies — 100 or more plasmids — can be present in a single bacterium, thus providing gene amplification.

This research on microorganisms bears enormous potential for future attack on human genetic disease at the DNA or genotype level. More immediately, genetic engineering may provide human gene products in an abundance never before even dreamed of. For example, in 1977 scientists chemically synthesized the gene for a precursor of human somatostatin, a 14-amino acid polypeptide hormone produced by the hypothalamus. The synthetic gene was introduced into *E. coli*, and 100 g of these bacteria growing in eight liters of culture medium produced 5 mg of the hormone. A similar amount of hormone had previously been isolated from the brains of one-half million sheep!

Genetic engineering should not be confused with science-fiction scenarios now being promulgated in the lay press. The creation of vertebrate monsters, or the programmed reproduction of identical men for political, economic, or military purposes are neither within the present possibilities nor future promises of genetic engineering. Some of the misconceptions stem from the public's mentally confusing DNA experiments on the one hand with recent advances in human genetics, such as prenatal diagnosis or artificial insemination on the other. Other misconceptions perhaps stem from words newly coined in genetic engineering but having well-established earlier connotations. Thus a *chimera* is joined DNA of two species, not the fire-breathing monster of Greek mythology. A *clone* is simply a selected colony of bacteria carrying a fragment of DNA in a plasmid vehicle enabling the DNA fragment to be reproduced. Such clones are unrelated to publicized but fictitious attempts to asexually reproduce human beings. A *hybrid* is a bacterium with perhaps one to 10 of its 4000 genes derived from another organism, not a half-and-half genetic mixture of man and bacterium or of man and mouse (Mickey Mouse?).

The diversity of successful therapeutic approaches to genetic disease and the new possibilities emerging from fundamental studies allow some optimism for the future.

Selected Reading

GENERAL

Bodmer WF, Cavalli-Sforza LL: Genetics, Evolution, and Man. San Francisco, WH Freeman & Co, 1976

Levitan M, Montagu A: Textbook of Human Genetics, ed 2. London, Oxford University Press, 1977

McKusick VA, Claiborne R (eds): Medical Genetics. New York, HP Publishing Co, 1973

Riccardi VM: The Genetic Approach to Human Disease. New York, Oxford University Press, 1977

Roberts JAF, Pembrey ME: An Introduction to Medical Genetics, ed 7. London, Oxford University Press, 1978

Stern C: Principles of Human Genetics, ed 3. San Francisco, WH Freeman & Co, 1973

Thompson JS, Thompson MW: Genetics in Medicine, ed 3. Philadelphia, WB Saunders Co, 1978

CYTOGENETICS

de Grouchy J, Turleau C: Clinical Atlas of Human Chromosomes. New York, John Wiley & Sons, 1977

McKusick VA, Ruddle FH: The status of the gene map of the human chromosomes. Science 196:390–405, 1977

Wachtel SS: H-Y antigen and the genetics of sex determination. Science 198:797–799, 1977

Witkin HA, Mednick SA, Schulsinger F, et al: Criminality in XYY and XXY men. Science 193:547–555, 1976

Yunis JJ: High resolution of human chromosomes. Science 191:1268–1270, 1976

MENDELIAN GENETICS

Harris H: The Principles of Human Biochemical Genetics, ed 2. Amsterdam, North-Holland, 1975
McKusick VA: Mendelian Inheritance in Man, ed 5. Baltimore, The Johns Hopkins Press, 1978
Milunsky A, Annar GJ (eds): Genetics and the Law. New York, Plenum Press, 1976
Stanbury JB, Wyngaarden JB, Frederickson DS: The Metabolic Basis of Inherited Disease, ed 4. New York, McGraw-Hill, 1978

ASSOCIATIONS OF GENETIC MARKERS AND DISEASES

Calin A, Fries JF: Striking prevalence of ankylosing spondylitis in "healthy" W27 positive males and females. N Engl J Med 293:835–839, 1975
Jackson JF, Currier RD, Terasaki PI, Morton NE: Spinocerebellar ataxia and HLA linkage. N Engl J Med 296:1138–1141, 1977
McMichael A, McDevitt H: The association between the HLA system and disease, in Steinberg AG, Bearn AG, Motulsky AG, et al (eds): Progress in Medical Genetics. Philadelphia, WB Saunders Co, 1977, vol 2
Neel JV: The genetics of juvenile-onset-type diabetes mellitus. N Engl J Med 297:1062–1063, 1977
Rosenberg LE, Kidd KK: HLA and disease susceptibility: a primer. N Engl J Med 297:1060–1062, 1977
Simon M, Bourel M, Genetet B, et al: Idiopathic hemochromatosis. Demonstration of recessive transmission and early detection by family HLA typing. N Engl J Med 297:1017–1021, 1977

POLYGENIC OR MULTIFACTORIAL GENETICS

Carter CO: Multifactorial genetic disease, in McKusick VA, Claiborne R (eds): Medical Genetics. New York, HP Publishing Co, 1973
Goodwin DW: Hereditary factors in alcoholism. Hospital Practice, May 1978, pp 121–130
Heston LL: Schizophrenia: genetic factors. Hospital Practice, June 1977, pp 43-49

BIOCHEMISTRY OF GENETIC EXPRESSION

Kornberg A: DNA Synthesis. San Francisco, WH Freeman & Co, 1974
Nienhuis AW, Benz EJ Jr: Regulation of hemoglobin sythesis during the development of the red cell. N Engl J Med 297:1318–1328 and 1371–1381, 1977
Orkin SH, Nathan DG: Current concepts in genetics. The Thalassemias. N Engl J Med 295:710–714, 1976
Watson JD: Molecular Biology of the Gene, ed 3. New York, WA Benjamin, 1976

GENETICS AND CANCER

Bergsma D (ed): Cancer and Genetics. Birth Defects: Original Article Series. New York, Alan R Liss, Inc, 1976, vol 12, no. 1
Fialkow PJ: The origin and development of human tumors studied with cell markers. N Engl J Med 291:26–35, 1974
Green M: Viral cell transformation in human oncogenesis. Hospital Practice, September 1975, pp 91–104
Jones KW: Chromosomes and malignancy. Nature 252:525, 1974
Mulvihill JJ, Miller RW, Fraumeni JF (eds): Genetics of Human Cancer. Progress in Cancer Research and Therapy. New York, Raven Press, 1977, vol 3
Rosen FR: Lymphoma, immunodeficiency, and the Epstein-Barr virus. N Engl J Med 297:1120–1121, 1977

TREATMENT OF GENETIC DISEASES

Aminocentesis Study Group: Midtrimester aminocentesis for prenatal diagnosis; safety and accuracy. JAMA 236:1471–1476, 1976
Blass JP, Gibson GE: Abnormality of a thiamine-requiring enzyme in patients with Wernicke-Korsakoff syndrome. N Engl J Med 297:1367–1370, 1977
Cohen SN: Recombinant DNA: fact and fiction. Science 195:654–657, 1977
Epstein CJ, Golbus MS: Prenatal diagnosis of genetic diseases. Am Scientist 65:703–711, 1977
Fuhrmann W, Vogel F: Genetic Counseling, ed 2. New York, Springer-Verlag, 1976
Kelly PT: Dealing with Dilemma. A Manual for Genetic Counselors. New York, Springer-Verlag, 1977
Stanbury JB, Wyngaarden JB, Frederickson DS: The Metabolic Basis of Inherited Disease, ed 4. New York, McGraw-Hill, 1978

INDEX